Pharmacoinformatics Real-World Applications in Pharmacy and Medicine

Mr. Prakash Nathaniel Kumar Sarella

Ms. Golla Venkata Sowmyasree

Dr. Soujanya Akkineni

Dr. Jaya Vasavi Gurrala

Dr. V. Rakshana

Dr. Averineni Ravi Kumar

Dr. Pamidi Lakshmi Prasanna

Mrs. Chollangi Bhargavi

Mrs. Meenakshi Tyagi

Dr. Syed Afzal Uddin Biyabani

ISBN: 978-81-979731-0-9

Pharmacoinformatics: Real-World Applications in Pharmacy and Medicine

By

Mr. Prakash Nathaniel Kumar Sarella

Dr. Averineni Ravi Kumar

Ms. Golla Venkata Sowmyasree

Dr. Pamidi Lakshmi Prasanna

Dr. Soujanya Akkineni

Mrs. Chollangi Bhargavi

Dr. Jaya Vasavi Gurrala

Mrs. Meenakshi Tyagi

Dr. V. Rakshana

Dr. Syed Afzal Uddin Biyabani

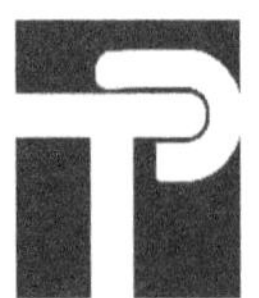

Copyright © 2024 ThinkPlus Pharma Publications

All rights reserved.

ISBN: 978-81-979731-0-9

DEDICATION

To all the healthcare professionals who tirelessly dedicate their lives to improving the well-being of others:
This book is a tribute to your unwavering commitment, compassion, and resilience. As pharmacists, physicians, and healthcare practitioners, you consistently go above and beyond to provide the best possible care for your patients, often in the face of unprecedented challenges and complexities.

In the rapidly evolving healthcare field, where technology and data play an increasingly crucial role, we recognize the importance of equipping you with the tools and knowledge necessary to harness the power of programming in your noble pursuit of better patient outcomes.

We dedicate this book to you, the unsung heroes who work tirelessly behind the scenes to ensure the health and safety of our communities. Your relentless pursuit of knowledge, your adaptability in the face of change, and your willingness to embrace new skills and technologies are truly inspiring.

CONTENTS

ACKNOWLEDGMENTS

We would like to express our deepest gratitude to all those who have contributed to the development and completion of this book, "Pharmacoinformatics: Real-World Applications in Pharmacy and Medicine." First, we would like to thank our families and friends for their unwavering support, patience, and understanding throughout the writing process. Your love and encouragement have been the driving force behind our dedication to this project.

We extend our sincere appreciation to the management and colleagues at our respective institutions and organizations. Your support, resources, and collaborative efforts have been invaluable in shaping the content and direction of this book. We are grateful for the opportunity to work alongside such knowledgeable and passionate professionals in the field of pharmacology.

Special thanks go to our editorial team, whose expertise and guidance have been instrumental in refining the structure, clarity, and accuracy of the book. Your attention to detail and commitment to excellence have elevated the quality of this work.

We also want to acknowledge the countless healthcare professionals, researchers, and educators who have contributed to the field of pharmacology. Your tireless efforts and groundbreaking discoveries have laid the foundation upon which this book is built.

Finally, we would like to thank our readers for their interest in "Pharmacoinformatics: Real-World Applications in Pharmacy and Medicine." We hope that this book will serve as a valuable resource in your pursuit of knowledge and excellence in patient care

.

PREFACE

The field of healthcare is undergoing a rapid digital transformation, and programming skills have become increasingly essential for professionals in this domain. As healthcare data continues to grow in volume and complexity, the ability to leverage programming languages and tools to analyze, interpret, and utilize this data effectively is crucial for driving innovation, improving patient outcomes, and optimizing healthcare delivery.

This book, "Pharmacoinformatics: Real-World Applications in Pharmacy and Medicine" is designed to bridge the gap between medicine and computer science by providing a practical and accessible introduction to programming languages and techniques specifically tailored to the needs of healthcare professionals. Whether you are a student, a practicing pharmacist, a physician, or any other healthcare professional, this book aims to equip you with the fundamental programming skills and domain-specific knowledge required to tackle real-world challenges in healthcare.

The book covers a wide range of programming languages and their applications in healthcare, including Python, R, Java, C++, SQL, and MATLAB. It is structured in a way that allows readers to gradually build their programming skills, starting from the basics and progressing to more advanced topics and case studies

PART I: INTRODUCTION TO PROGRAMMING FOR HEALTHCARE

1 THE IMPORTANCE OF PROGRAMMING IN PHARMACY AND MEDICINE

The field of healthcare is undergoing a remarkable transformation, and at the heart of this change lies the growing importance of programming. As technology continues to advance at an unprecedented pace, healthcare professionals in pharmacy and medicine are increasingly recognizing the vital role that programming plays in their day-to-day work and the overall advancement of their respective fields.

Programming has become an essential tool in the modern healthcare toolkit, offering a wide range of benefits and applications that are transforming the way we approach patient care, research, and decision-making. It is no longer a niche skill reserved for IT professionals; rather, it has become a fundamental competency that every healthcare professional should strive to acquire.

One of the most significant advantages of programming in pharmacy and medicine is its ability to streamline processes and optimize workflows. In the fast-paced and often complex world of healthcare, efficiency is paramount.

Healthcare professionals are constantly seeking ways to simplify tasks, reduce errors, and improve overall productivity. This is where programming comes into play.

Pharmacists and physicians can automate repetitive and time-consuming tasks, freeing up valuable time and resources that can be better spent on patient care by developing custom software solutions tailored to their specific needs. For example, a well-designed medication management system can revolutionize the way pharmacists handle prescription orders, inventory tracking, and patient communication. Such a system can automatically generate accurate dispensing labels, send refill reminders to patients, and even flag potential drug interactions, thereby reducing the risk of medication errors and enhancing patient safety.

Similarly, in the realm of medical practice, programming can help streamline electronic health record (EHR) management, appointment scheduling, and billing processes. Physicians can focus more on providing quality care to their patients and less on paperwork and bureaucracy by automating these administrative tasks.

Another crucial aspect of programming in healthcare is its role in data analysis and interpretation. In today's data-driven world, healthcare professionals are inundated with vast amounts of information from various sources, including EHRs, wearable devices, and clinical trials. Making sense of this data and extracting meaningful insights is a daunting task, but one that programming can greatly facilitate.

Through the use of data analysis techniques and machine learning algorithms, healthcare professionals can harness the power of big data to identify patterns, predict patient outcomes, and make informed decisions. For instance, by analyzing patient data from EHRs, pharmacists can identify individuals who are at high risk of medication non-adherence and develop targeted interventions to improve their adherence rates. Similarly, physicians can use predictive modeling to identify patients who are most likely to benefit from a particular treatment, enabling them to provide personalized care that optimizes patient outcomes.

Programming also plays a pivotal role in advancing

healthcare research. From drug discovery and development to clinical trial design and analysis, programming tools and techniques have become indispensable in the quest for scientific breakthroughs. Researchers rely on programming to process large datasets, perform complex statistical analyses, and create sophisticated models that simulate biological processes and predict drug interactions.

For example, in the field of drug discovery, programming enables researchers to screen vast libraries of compounds and identify potential drug candidates more efficiently than ever before. Researchers can predict the binding affinity of a drug to its target protein, by using machine learning algorithms and molecular dynamics simulations, accelerating the drug discovery process and bringing new treatments to patients faster.

In clinical trials, programming is essential for designing robust study protocols, managing patient data, and analyzing trial results. With the help of programming, researchers can ensure data integrity, detect potential biases, and draw valid conclusions from their studies. This, in turn, helps to advance medical knowledge and inform evidence-based practice.

Programming is also at the forefront of the personalized medicine revolution. As we move towards a more individualized approach to healthcare, programming is enabling the development of algorithms and decision support systems that can tailor treatments to a patient's unique genetic profile, lifestyle factors, and medical history. These systems can generate personalized treatment recommendations that optimize efficacy and minimize adverse effects by integrating patient-specific data and applying machine learning techniques.

Moreover, programming is driving the development of innovative healthcare technologies that are transforming the way we deliver care. From mobile health apps that enable remote monitoring and patient engagement to telemedicine platforms that connect patients with healthcare providers across distances, programming is the driving force behind these groundbreaking solutions.

As healthcare professionals, it is crucial to recognize the importance of programming and actively engage in its application. Pharmacists and physicians can help shape the development of user-friendly and clinically relevant tools by acquiring programming skills and collaborating with technology experts that meet the needs of both patients and practitioners.

Moreover, programming skills are becoming increasingly valuable for effective communication and collaboration in the modern healthcare setting. As healthcare becomes more interdisciplinary and data-driven, the ability to speak the language of technology and work seamlessly with professionals from diverse backgrounds is essential. healthcare professionals can bridge the gap between clinical expertise and technical knowledge, fostering a culture of innovation and driving the development of more effective healthcare solutions by understanding the fundamentals of programming.

2 OVERVIEW OF PROGRAMMING LANGUAGES RELEVANT TO HEALTHCARE

In the rapidly evolving healthcare field, various programming languages have emerged as powerful tools for tackling the unique challenges and opportunities presented by this field. From data analysis and machine learning to software development and scientific computing, each language brings its own set of strengths and capabilities to the table. Programming languages that have proven particularly relevant and valuable in the context of healthcare: Python, R, Java, C++, SQL, MATLAB, Rust, Julia, Swift, and Go.

Python has become one of the most popular programming languages in healthcare, thanks to its simplicity, versatility, and extensive ecosystem of libraries and frameworks. Its clean syntax and readability make it an ideal choice for beginners and experienced programmers alike. In healthcare, Python is widely used for data analysis, machine learning, and the development of web applications and decision support systems. Libraries such as NumPy, Pandas, and Scikit-learn provide powerful tools for handling and analyzing large datasets, while frameworks like Django and Flask facilitate the creation of robust and scalable web applications.

R, on the other hand, is a language specifically designed for statistical computing and graphics. It has gained significant traction in the healthcare domain, particularly in the areas of biostatistics, epidemiology, and clinical research. R offers a wide range of statistical and graphical techniques, making it an essential tool for data visualization, hypothesis testing, and predictive modeling. Packages like ggplot2, dplyr, and tidyr streamline the process of data manipulation and visualization, while libraries such as Bioconductor provide extensive resources for bioinformatics and genomic data analysis.

Java is a general-purpose, object-oriented programming language that has found wide adoption in healthcare software development. Its platform independence, robustness, and scalability make it well-suited for building enterprise-level applications and systems. In healthcare, Java is commonly used for developing electronic health record (EHR) systems, clinical decision support tools, and telemedicine platforms. Frameworks such as Spring and Hibernate simplify the development process and promote code reusability, while libraries like Apache Spark and Flink enable high-performance data processing and analytics.

C++ is a powerful, high-performance language that is often used in healthcare when speed and efficiency are paramount. Its ability to provide low-level control over system resources makes it an ideal choice for developing performance-critical applications, such as medical imaging software, biosignal processing algorithms, and real-time monitoring systems. C++ also finds use in computational biology and bioinformatics, where its performance characteristics are valuable for handling large-scale genomic data and complex simulations.

SQL (Structured Query Language) is the standard language for managing and manipulating relational databases. In healthcare, SQL plays a crucial role in storing, retrieving, and analyzing patient data, electronic health records, and clinical trial information. SQL supports data-driven decision-making and facilitates the integration of disparate healthcare systems by enabling efficient data management and complex querying,. Database management systems like MySQL, PostgreSQL, and Microsoft SQL Server are widely used in healthcare organizations to ensure data integrity, security, and accessibility.

MATLAB (MATrix LABoratory) is a proprietary

programming language and numerical computing environment that is extensively used in healthcare research and development. Its strengths lie in matrix manipulations, signal and image processing, and algorithm development. MATLAB's built-in functions and toolboxes provide a rich set of tools for tasks such as medical image analysis, biosignal processing, and computational modeling. It is particularly popular in fields like medical imaging, neuroscience, and biomedical engineering, where its interactive environment and visualization capabilities accelerate the development and testing of new algorithms and techniques.

Rust is a systems programming language that prioritizes safety, concurrency, and memory efficiency. Although relatively new compared to other languages, Rust has gained attention in healthcare for its potential to build secure and reliable software systems. Its strong static typing, ownership system, and thread safety guarantees make it well-suited for developing mission-critical applications, such as medical device software, clinical decision support systems, and telemedicine platforms. Rust's growing ecosystem of libraries and frameworks, such as the Rust-Bio project, also makes it an attractive choice for bioinformatics and computational biology tasks.

Julia is a high-level, high-performance dynamic programming language designed for numerical and scientific computing. It combines the ease of use and expressiveness of Python with the performance of C++, making it an attractive option for healthcare applications that require both simplicity and speed. Julia's ability to seamlessly integrate with other languages, such as C and Fortran, allows it to leverage existing libraries and codebases. In healthcare, Julia finds applications in areas like computational biology, pharmacometrics, and health economics, where its performance and flexibility are highly valued.

Swift is a modern, fast, and safe programming language developed by Apple for iOS, macOS, and other Apple platforms. While primarily used for developing mobile and desktop applications, Swift has also gained traction in healthcare app development. Its expressive syntax, strong typing, and extensive standard library make it a productive language for creating user-friendly and secure healthcare applications. Swift's integration with Apple's healthcare frameworks, such as HealthKit and CareKit, simplifies the development of apps that leverage health data and promote patient engagement.

Go, also known as Golang, is a statically typed, compiled language developed by Google. It offers simplicity, efficiency, and built-in support for concurrency, making it well-suited for building scalable and performant backend systems. In healthcare, Go is gaining popularity for developing microservices, APIs, and data processing pipelines. Its lightweight runtime and low memory footprint make it an attractive choice for cloud-based healthcare solutions and IoT applications. Go's standard library and growing ecosystem of healthcare-related packages, such as FHIR (Fast Healthcare Interoperability Resources) clients and HL7 parsers, further enhance its utility in the healthcare domain.

Each of these programming languages brings unique strengths and capabilities to the healthcare field. Python and R excel in data analysis and machine learning, while Java and C++ are well-suited for building robust and efficient software systems. SQL is essential for managing and querying healthcare databases, and MATLAB is a go-to choice for medical research and algorithm development. Rust and Julia offer new possibilities for building secure and high-performance applications, while Swift and Go are making inroads in mobile app development and backend systems, respectively.

3 SETTING UP YOUR PROGRAMMING ENVIRONMENT

Before diving into the exciting world of healthcare programming, it is essential to set up a proper development environment. This involves installing and configuring the necessary tools, such as Integrated Development Environments (IDEs) and package managers, which will streamline your workflow and make your programming experience more efficient and enjoyable. In this chapter, we will guide you through the process of setting up your programming environment, focusing on installing and configuring IDEs and exploring package managers and libraries

3.1 Installing and Configuring IDEs

An IDE is a software application that provides a comprehensive environment for writing, debugging, and testing code. It combines a text editor, compiler, debugger, and other tools into a single graphical user interface, making it easier to develop and manage your programming projects. While it is possible to write code using a simple text editor, IDEs offer a range of features that enhance productivity and make the development process more intuitive.

When choosing an IDE, consider factors such as the programming languages you will be working with, the platform you are developing for, and your personal preferences in terms of user interface and functionality. Some popular IDEs for healthcare programming include:

Visual Studio Code: A lightweight, cross-platform IDE developed by Microsoft that supports a wide range of programming languages, including Python, R, Java, and C++. It offers a rich ecosystem of extensions, making it highly customizable to suit your specific needs.

PyCharm: A powerful IDE for Python development, created by JetBrains. It provides intelligent code completion, code inspections, and integrated debugging tools, making it a popular choice for data analysis and machine learning projects in healthcare.

RStudio: An IDE specifically designed for R programming. It offers a user-friendly interface, interactive console, and integrated plotting and debugging tools, making it the go-to choice for statistical computing and data visualization in healthcare research.

Eclipse: A versatile, open-source IDE that supports multiple programming languages, including Java, C++, and Python. Its extensive plugin system allows you to customize the environment to your liking, making it suitable for a wide range of healthcare software development projects.

Xcode: Apple's official IDE for developing applications for macOS, iOS, and other Apple platforms. It provides a comprehensive set of tools for Swift and Objective-C development, making it the primary choice for creating healthcare apps for Apple devices.

Once you have selected an IDE, the installation process is usually straightforward. Most IDEs provide downloadable installers or packages that guide you through the setup process. During installation, you may be prompted to choose the components or plugins you want to include, depending on your specific requirements.

After installation, take some time to familiarize yourself with the IDE's interface and customize it to your preferences. This may involve adjusting the color scheme, font size, and keyboard shortcuts, or installing additional plugins and extensions to enhance functionality.

3.2 Package Managers and Libraries

Package managers are tools that simplify the process of installing, updating, and managing software packages and libraries. They automate the retrieval and installation of dependencies, ensuring that your projects have access to the necessary libraries and modules without the need for manual setup.

Each programming language has its own package management system, and familiarizing yourself with the relevant tools is crucial for efficient development. Some popular package managers include:

1. *pip:* The standard package manager for Python. It allows you to easily install and manage Python packages and their dependencies. With a simple command like pip install numpy, you can install the NumPy library, which is widely used for numerical computing in healthcare data analysis.

2. *conda:* An open-source package management system and environment management system for Python and R. It provides a streamlined way to install and manage packages, as well as create isolated environments for different projects. Conda is particularly useful when working with data science and machine learning libraries like Scikit-learn and TensorFlow.

3. *CRAN (Comprehensive R Archive Network):* The primary repository for R packages. It hosts a wide range of packages contributed by the R community, covering various domains such as statistical analysis, data visualization, and bioinformatics. Installing packages in R is as simple as running install.packages("ggplot2") to install the popular data visualization library ggplot2.

4. *Maven and Gradle:* Build automation and dependency management tools for Java projects. They simplify the process of managing external libraries and ensure that your projects have access to the required dependencies. These tools are commonly used in Java-based healthcare software

development projects.

5. npm (Node Package Manager): The default package manager for JavaScript and Node.js. While primarily used for web development, npm also hosts packages relevant to healthcare, such as the fhir.js library for working with FHIR (Fast Healthcare Interoperability Resources) data.

In addition to package managers, it's important to familiarize yourself with the standard libraries and frameworks associated with each programming language. These libraries provide a foundation for building healthcare applications and offer pre-built functionality for common tasks.

For example, Python's standard library includes modules for file I/O, data structures, and networking, while specialized libraries like NumPy, Pandas, and Matplotlib are essential for data manipulation, analysis, and visualization in healthcare. Similarly, R's base packages provide a wide range of statistical and graphical functions, while libraries like dplyr and tidyr are indispensable for data wrangling and cleaning.

When working on healthcare projects, you'll often need to leverage domain-specific libraries and frameworks. These may include libraries for working with medical imaging data (e.g., SimpleITK for Python), bioinformatics toolkits (e.g., Bioconductor for R), or health information exchange standards (e.g., HAPI FHIR for Java). Familiarizing yourself with the relevant libraries and their documentation will greatly enhance your ability to tackle healthcare-specific programming challenges.

Setting up your programming environment is an essential step in your journey as a healthcare programmer. You'll be well-equipped to start building innovative solutions that can transform healthcare delivery and improve patient outcomes by installing and configuring the appropriate IDEs, package managers, and libraries. As you progress in your programming skills, don't hesitate to explore new tools and libraries that can further streamline your workflow and expand your capabilities. Remember, a well-organized and efficient programming environment is the foundation upon which you'll build the future of healthcare technology.

PART II: INTRODUCTION TO PROGRAMMING FOR HEALTHCARE

4 INTRODUCTION TO PYTHON PROGRAMMING

Python has emerged as one of the most popular and versatile programming languages in the healthcare industry. Its simplicity, readability, and extensive ecosystem of libraries make it an ideal choice for a wide range of healthcare applications, from data analysis and machine learning to software development and automation. In this chapter, we will dive into the fundamentals of Python programming, exploring its basic syntax and data types, setting the foundation for building powerful and efficient healthcare solutions.

4.1 Basic Syntax

Python's syntax is designed to be clean, concise, and intuitive, making it easy for beginners to learn and understand. Let's start by examining some of the key elements of Python's syntax.

4.1.1 Indentation: Unlike many other programming languages that use curly braces or keywords to define code blocks, Python relies on indentation. This means that the whitespace at the beginning of a line determines the grouping of statements. Typically, four spaces are used for each level of indentation, although the number of spaces can vary as long as it remains consistent within a code block. This enforced indentation helps maintain code readability and reduces the likelihood of syntax errors.

4.1.2 Comments: Comments are used to add explanatory notes or annotations within the code, making it easier for developers to understand and maintain. In Python, single-line comments start with the hash character (#), while multi-line comments are enclosed between triple quotes (""" or "). Comments are ignored by the Python interpreter and do not affect the execution of the code.

4.1.3 Variables: Variables are used to store and manipulate data in Python. Unlike some statically-typed languages, Python is dynamically-typed, meaning that you don't need to explicitly declare the type of a variable before using it. To assign a value to a variable, you simply use the equal sign (=) followed by the desired value. For example, age = 25 assigns the integer value 25 to the variable age.

4.1.4 Operators: Python supports a wide range of operators for performing arithmetic, comparison, and logical operations. Some common operators include + (addition), - (subtraction), * (multiplication), / (division), % (modulo), == (equality), != (inequality), < (less than), > (greater than), and (logical AND), and or (logical OR). These operators allow you to perform calculations, make comparisons, and control the flow of your program.

4.1.5 Control Flow: Python provides several control flow statements that allow you to govern the order in which code is executed based on certain conditions. The if, elif (else if), and else statements are used for conditional execution, allowing you to specify different code paths based on whether a condition is true or false. The for and while loops enable you to repeatedly execute a block of code until a specific condition is met, making it easy to perform iterations and process large datasets.

4.1.6 Functions: Functions are reusable blocks of code that perform a specific task. They help organize your code, improve readability, and promote code reuse. To define a function in Python, you use the def keyword followed by the function name, parentheses containing any input parameters, and a colon. The function body is indented below the definition line. Functions can optionally return a value using the return statement.

4.2 Data Types

Python provides a rich set of built-in data types that allow you to efficiently store and manipulate different kinds of data. Understanding these data types is crucial for working with healthcare data, which often includes numeric measurements, patient records, and medical terminology. Let's explore some of the fundamental data types in Python.

4.2.1 Numeric Types

Integer (int): Represents whole numbers, such as 42 or -10. Integers have unlimited precision, meaning they can store arbitrarily large numbers.

Float (float): Represents decimal numbers, such as 3.14 or -2.5. Floats are stored with a fixed precision, typically up to 15 decimal places.

Complex (complex): Represents complex numbers, consisting of a real and imaginary part, such as 2 + 3j. Complex numbers are useful in certain mathematical and scientific computations.

4.2.2 Boolean Type

Boolean (bool): Represents a truth value, either True or False. Booleans are commonly used in conditional statements and logical operations.

4.2.3 Sequence Types

String (str): Represents a sequence of characters, such as

"Hello, World!" or 'Python is awesome'. Strings are immutable, meaning they cannot be changed after creation. Python provides a wide range of string methods for manipulation and processing, such as lower(), upper(), split(), and join().

List (list): Represents an ordered collection of items, which can be of different types. Lists are mutable, allowing you to add, remove, or modify elements after creation. They are defined using square brackets, such as [1, 2, 3] or ['apple', 'banana', 'cherry']. Lists are widely used for storing and processing sequences of data in healthcare, such as patient records or time-series measurements.

Tuple (tuple): Represents an ordered, immutable collection of items, similar to lists. However, once a tuple is created, its elements cannot be changed. Tuples are defined using parentheses, such as (1, 2, 3) or ('red', 'green', 'blue'). Tuples are often used to store related pieces of data that should not be modified, such as patient demographics or medication dosages.

4.2.4 Mapping Type

Dictionary (dict): Represents an unordered collection of key-value pairs, where each key is unique. Dictionaries are mutable and allow efficient lookup and retrieval of values based on their keys. They are defined using curly braces, with keys and values separated by colons, such as {'name': 'John', 'age': 30, 'city': 'New York'}. Dictionaries are commonly used to store structured data, such as patient records or configuration settings.

4.2.5 Set Types

Set (set): Represents an unordered collection of unique elements. Sets are mutable and support operations like union, intersection, and difference. They are defined using curly braces or the set() constructor, such as {1, 2, 3} or set(['a', 'b', 'c']). Sets are useful for tasks like removing duplicates or checking for membership.

Frozen Set (frozenset): Represents an immutable version of a set. Frozen sets are hashable and can be used as keys in dictionaries or elements of other sets.

In addition to these built-in data types, Python also provides specialized data types through its extensive standard library and third-party packages. For example, the datetime module offers types for working with dates and times, while the NumPy library introduces high-performance multidimensional arrays and mathematical functions, which are essential for scientific computing and data analysis in healthcare.

As you progress in your Python programming journey, you'll encounter more advanced data types and structures, such as classes and objects, which allow you to define your own custom types and encapsulate related data and behavior. In the upcoming chapters, we will explore how to leverage these fundamental concepts to tackle real-world healthcare challenges, from analyzing patient data and developing predictive models to building interactive dashboards and automating clinical workflows.

Remember, practice is key to becoming proficient in Python programming. Don't hesitate to experiment with code snippets, explore the Python documentation, and seek guidance from the vibrant Python community.

4.3 Control Structures and Functions

Control structures and functions are fundamental building blocks in Python programming that allow you to control the flow of your code and organize it into reusable and modular components. Mastering these concepts is essential for writing efficient, readable, and maintainable Python code in healthcare applications. Let's dive into the details of control structures and functions in Python.

4.3.1 Control Structures

Control structures in Python enable you to make decisions and repeat code based on certain conditions. There are three main types of control structures: conditional statements, loops, and exception handling.

Conditional Statements:

if statement: The if statement allows you to execute a block of code only if a specified condition is true. It is used for decision-making and branching in your code.

if-else statement: The if-else statement extends the if statement by providing an alternative block of code to execute if the condition is false. It allows you to specify different actions based on the outcome of a condition.

if-elif-else statement: The if-elif-else statement allows you to chain multiple conditions together. It checks each condition in order and executes the block of code associated with the first true condition. If none of the conditions are true, the else block is executed.

4.3.2 Loops

for loop: The for loop is used to iterate over a sequence (such as a list, tuple, or string) or other iterable objects. It allows you to execute a block of code repeatedly for each item in the sequence.

while loop: The while loop repeatedly executes a block of code as long as a given condition is true. It is useful when you don't know the exact number of iterations in advance and want to continue executing until a certain condition is met.

Loop control statements:

break: The break statement allows you to exit a loop prematurely, even if the loop condition is still true. It is commonly used to handle special cases or to terminate the loop based on a specific condition.

continue: The continue statement allows you to skip the rest of the current iteration and move to the next iteration of the loop. It is useful when you want to ignore certain items or conditions within the loop.

4.3.3 Exception Handling

try-except statement: The try-except statement is used to handle exceptions (errors) that may occur during the execution of your code. It allows you to gracefully handle and recover from exceptions, preventing your program from abruptly terminating.

try-except-else statement: The try-except-else statement extends the try-except statement by providing an optional else block that is executed if no exceptions occur within the try block.

try-except-finally statement: The try-except-finally statement adds a finally block to the try-except statement. The finally block is executed regardless of whether an exception occurs or not, making it useful for cleanup tasks or releasing resources.

4.4 Functions

Functions in Python are reusable blocks of code that perform a specific task. They help in organizing code, improving readability, and promoting code reuse. Functions can take input parameters, perform computations or actions, and optionally return a value.

4.4.1. Defining Functions:

Function declaration: To define a function in Python, you use the def keyword followed by the function name, parentheses containing any input parameters, and a colon. The function body is indented below the definition line.

Function parameters: Functions can accept input parameters, which are values passed to the function when it is called. Parameters allow you to provide data to the function for processing or customization.

Default parameter values: Python allows you to specify default values for function parameters. If an argument is not provided when calling the function, the default value is used instead.

Returning values: Functions can optionally return a value using the return statement. The returned value can be captured and used by the caller of the function.

4.4.2 Calling Functions

Function invocation: To execute a function, you simply call it by its name followed by parentheses containing any required arguments. The function's code block is executed, and any returned value can be captured.

Argument passing: When calling a function, you can pass arguments to it in the same order as the function's parameter list. Python supports positional arguments, keyword arguments, and a combination of both.

4.4.3. Variable Scope:

Local variables: Variables defined within a function have a local scope, meaning they are only accessible within the function. Local variables are created when the function is called and destroyed when the function exits.

Global variables: Variables defined outside any function have a global scope and can be accessed from anywhere in the code, including inside functions. However, if you want to modify a global variable within a function, you need to use the global keyword to indicate that you are referring to the global variable.

4.4.4 Recursive Functions

Recursion: Python supports recursive functions, which are functions that call themselves within their own code block. Recursion is a powerful technique for solving problems that can be divided into smaller subproblems.

Base case: In recursive functions, it's crucial to define a base case that specifies the condition under which the recursion should stop. The base case prevents infinite recursion and allows the function to eventually return a result.

4.5 Object-Oriented Programming (OOP) in Python

Object-oriented programming is a programming paradigm that organizes code into objects, which are instances of classes. It promotes code modularity, reusability, and encapsulation. Python provides robust support for OOP, making it easy to create and work with classes and objects.

4.5.1 Classes

Class definition: A class is a blueprint or template for creating objects. It defines the attributes (data) and methods (functions) that the objects of the class will have. In Python, you define a class using the class keyword followed by the class name and a colon.

Attributes: Attributes are the data members of a class. They represent the state or properties of an object. Attributes can be defined within the class or initialized in the constructor method.

Methods: Methods are the functions associated with a class. They define the behavior or actions that objects of the class can perform. Methods are defined within the class and can access and manipulate the object's attributes.

Constructor: The constructor is a special method called __init__() that is automatically called when creating a new object. It is used to initialize the object's attributes and perform any necessary setup.

4.5.2 Objects

Object creation: Objects are instances of a class. They are created by calling the class name as if it were a function, which invokes the constructor to initialize the object.

Object attributes: Each object has its own set of attribute values, which can be accessed and modified using dot notation (e.g., object.attribute).

Object methods: Objects can call the methods defined in their class using dot notation (e.g., object.method()). Methods operate on the object's attributes and perform specific actions.

4.5.3. Inheritance

Inheritance: Inheritance is a mechanism that allows a class to inherit attributes and methods from another class, called the superclass or base class. The class that inherits is called the subclass or derived class. Inheritance promotes code reuse and allows for the creation of specialized classes based on existing ones.

Single inheritance: Python supports single inheritance, where a subclass inherits from a single superclass. The subclass inherits all the attributes and methods of the superclass and can add its own specific attributes and methods.

Multiple inheritance: Python also supports multiple inheritance, where a subclass can inherit from multiple superclasses. The subclass inherits attributes and methods from all its superclasses, allowing for the combination of functionalities from different classes.

4.5.4 Polymorphism

Polymorphism: Polymorphism refers to the ability of objects of different classes to respond to the same method call in different ways. It allows for flexibility and extensibility in object-oriented design.

Method overriding: Method overriding occurs when a subclass defines a method with the same name as a method in its superclass. The subclass's method overrides the superclass's method, providing a specialized implementation.

Method overloading: Python does not support method overloading in the same way as some other programming languages. However, you can achieve similar functionality by using default parameter values or by defining methods with different parameter types.

4.5.5. Encapsulation

Encapsulation: Encapsulation is the principle of bundling data (attributes) and methods that operate on that data within a class. It helps in achieving data protection and maintaining the integrity of an object's state.

Access modifiers: Python does not have strict access modifiers like some other programming languages. However, by convention, attributes and methods that are intended to be private or protected are prefixed with an underscore (_) or double underscore (__), respectively.

Object-oriented programming is particularly useful in healthcare applications, as it allows for the creation of modular and reusable code components. For example, you can define classes for patients, medical records, medications, and clinical procedures, each with their own attributes and methods. OOP facilitates the organization and management of complex healthcare data and logic, making the code more maintainable and scalable.

When designing classes and objects in healthcare applications, consider the following best practices:

1. Encapsulate related data and behavior within classes to promote modularity and cohesion.
2. Use inheritance to create specialized classes based on common base classes, promoting code reuse and extensibility.
3. Utilize polymorphism to define common interfaces and allow for flexible interactions between objects.
4. Follow naming conventions and use meaningful names for classes, attributes, and methods to enhance code readability.
5. Implement appropriate access control and data protection mechanisms to ensure the security of healthcare data.

5 DATA ANALYSIS AND VISUALIZATION WITH PYTHON

Data analysis and visualization are crucial aspects of healthcare informatics, as they enable practitioners and researchers to extract valuable insights from vast amounts of medical data. Python provides a rich ecosystem of libraries and tools specifically designed for data manipulation, analysis, and visualization. In this chapter, we will explore two fundamental libraries: NumPy and Pandas, which form the backbone of data analysis workflows in Python.

5.1 NumPy for Numerical Computing

NumPy (Numerical Python) is a powerful library that provides support for large, multi-dimensional arrays and matrices, along with a collection of mathematical functions to operate on these arrays efficiently. It is the foundation upon which many other data analysis and scientific computing libraries are built.

5.1.1 NumPy Arrays

Creating arrays: NumPy arrays can be created using various methods, such as np.array(), np.zeros(), np.ones(), np.arange(), and np.linspace(). These functions allow you to create arrays with specific values, shapes, and data types.

Array attributes: NumPy arrays have several important attributes, including shape (dimensions of the array), dtype (data type of the elements), and size (total number of elements).

Indexing and slicing: NumPy arrays support efficient indexing and slicing operations, allowing you to access and manipulate specific elements or subsets of the array.

5.1.2 Mathematical Operations

Element-wise operations: NumPy enables element-wise operations on arrays, such as addition, subtraction, multiplication, and division. These operations are performed efficiently, without the need for explicit loops.

Broadcasting: NumPy's broadcasting feature allows arrays with different shapes to be used in arithmetic operations, as long as their dimensions are compatible. This simplifies code and improves performance.

Mathematical functions: NumPy provides a wide range of mathematical functions that can be applied element-wise to arrays, such as trigonometric functions (np.sin(), np.cos()), exponential and logarithmic functions (np.exp(), np.log()), and statistical functions (np.mean(), np.std()).

5.1.3 Array Manipulation

Reshaping arrays: NumPy allows you to change the shape of an array using functions like reshape(), flatten(), and transpose(). This is useful when you need to adapt the array's structure to match the requirements of a particular operation or algorithm.

Combining arrays: NumPy provides functions to concatenate arrays (np.concatenate()), stack arrays vertically or horizontally (np.vstack(), np.hstack()), and split arrays into smaller subarrays (np.split(), np.hsplit(), np.vsplit()).

Boolean indexing and masking: NumPy supports boolean indexing, which allows you to select elements from an array based on a boolean condition. This is particularly useful for filtering and selecting specific subsets of data.

5.2 Pandas for Data Manipulation

Pandas is a powerful data manipulation library built on top of NumPy. It introduces two primary data structures: Series and DataFrame, which provide a convenient way to work with structured and labeled data.

5.2.1 Series

Creating Series: A Series is a one-dimensional labeled array that can hold any data type. It can be created from a list, NumPy array, or dictionary using the pd.Series() function.

Series attributes: Series have attributes such as values (the underlying data), index (the labels associated with each element), and dtype (the data type of the elements).

Indexing and slicing: Series support efficient indexing and slicing operations based on their labels or integer positions.

5.2.2 DataFrame

Creating DataFrames: A DataFrame is a two-dimensional labeled data structure, similar to a spreadsheet or SQL table. It consists of rows and columns, where each column can have a different data type. DataFrames can be created from various sources, such as lists, dictionaries, NumPy arrays, or external files (CSV, Excel, SQL databases).

DataFrame attributes: DataFrames have attributes like columns (the column labels), index (the row labels), shape (the dimensions of the DataFrame), and dtypes (the data types of each column).

Indexing and selection: DataFrames provide flexible indexing and selection operations, allowing you to access specific rows, columns, or subsets of the data using labels or boolean conditions.

5.2.3 Data Manipulation

Filtering and sorting: Pandas enables filtering rows based on conditions using boolean indexing or the loc[] and iloc[] accessors. You can also sort the DataFrame by one or more columns using the sort_values() function.

Merging and joining: Pandas provides functions to merge and join DataFrames based on common columns or indexes, similar to SQL joins. This allows you to combine data from multiple sources or perform database-like operations on DataFrames.

Grouping and aggregation: Pandas supports grouping data by one or more columns using the groupby() function. You can then apply aggregation functions (e.g., sum, mean, count) to each group, enabling powerful data summarization and analysis.

Handling missing data: Pandas offers functions to detect and handle missing data, such as isnull(), dropna(), and fillna(). These functions allow you to identify missing values, remove rows or columns with missing data, or fill in missing values with specified values or interpolation methods.

5.3 Applications of NumPy and Pandas

In the context of healthcare data analysis, NumPy and Pandas are invaluable tools for processing and analyzing medical datasets. Here are a few examples of how these libraries can be applied:

5.3.1 Patient Data Analysis

Using Pandas, you can load patient data from various sources (e.g., CSV files, SQL databases) into a DataFrame, allowing for easy exploration and manipulation.

You can filter and select specific subsets of patients based on criteria such as age, gender, or medical conditions using boolean indexing or the loc[] and iloc[] accessors.

Pandas enables merging and joining patient data from different sources, such as combining demographic information with clinical records or laboratory results.

You can perform grouping and aggregation operations to calculate summary statistics, such as the average age of patients with a specific condition or the prevalence of certain symptoms across different patient groups.

5.3.2 Medical Image Processing

NumPy arrays are commonly used to represent and

process medical images, such as MRI scans, CT scans, or X-rays.

You can perform element-wise operations on image arrays, such as applying filters, normalizing pixel values, or performing mathematical transformations.

NumPy's indexing and slicing capabilities allow you to extract specific regions of interest (ROIs) from medical images for further analysis or visualization.

Libraries like scikit-image and OpenCV, which are built on top of NumPy, provide additional functionalities for image processing tasks, such as segmentation, registration, and feature extraction.

5.3.3 Time Series Analysis

Pandas' DatetimeIndex and time series functionality make it well-suited for analyzing temporal healthcare data, such as patient monitoring data or disease progression over time.

You can resample time series data to different frequencies (e.g., hourly, daily, weekly) using the resample() function, enabling analysis at various time scales.

Pandas allows you to perform rolling window operations, such as calculating moving averages or detecting trends and anomalies in time series data.

You can align and synchronize time series data from multiple sources using Pandas' datetime alignment capabilities, facilitating the comparison and correlation of temporal patterns.

These are just a few examples of how NumPy and Pandas can be applied in healthcare data analysis. As you dive deeper into these libraries and explore their functionalities, you'll discover countless possibilities for manipulating, transforming, and extracting insights from medical datasets.

To further enhance your data analysis workflows, you can combine NumPy and Pandas with other powerful Python libraries, such as Matplotlib and Seaborn for data visualization, scikit-learn for machine learning, and SciPy for scientific computing. Together, these libraries form a comprehensive toolkit for tackling complex data analysis tasks in healthcare.

As you work with healthcare data using NumPy and Pandas, it's important to consider data privacy and security aspects. Ensure that you handle sensitive patient information in compliance with relevant regulations and guidelines, such as HIPAA (Health Insurance Portability and Accountability Act) in the United States or GDPR (General Data Protection Regulation) in the European Union.

5.4 Matplotlib and Seaborn for Data Visualization

Data visualization is an essential component of data analysis, as it allows you to communicate insights and patterns effectively to both technical and non-technical audiences. Python offers two powerful libraries for creating informative and visually appealing visualizations: Matplotlib and Seaborn. In this section, we will explore the capabilities of these libraries and how they can be used to visualize healthcare data.

5.4.1 Matplotlib

Matplotlib is a fundamental plotting library in Python that provides a wide range of functionalities for creating static, animated, and interactive visualizations. It offers low-level control over every aspect of a plot, allowing you to customize your visualizations extensively.

1. Basic Plotting

Line plots: Matplotlib allows you to create line plots using the plt.plot() function. You can specify the x and y coordinates of the data points, customize line styles, colors, and markers, and add labels and titles to the plot.

Scatter plots: Scatter plots are useful for visualizing the relationship between two variables. You can create scatter plots using the plt.scatter() function, where you provide the x and y coordinates of the data points. Matplotlib allows you to control the size, color, and transparency of the markers.

Bar plots: Bar plots are commonly used to compare categories or display the distribution of a variable. Matplotlib provides the plt.bar() and plt.barh() functions for creating vertical and horizontal bar plots, respectively. You can specify the heights or lengths of the bars, customize their colors and widths, and add labels and legends.

2. Subplots and Multiple Plots

Subplots: Matplotlib enables you to create multiple subplots within a single figure using the plt.subplots() function. This is useful when you want to display different visualizations side by side or in a grid layout. You can specify the number of rows and columns of subplots and access each subplot individually for further customization.

Multiple plots: You can also create multiple plots on the same axes using functions like plt.plot(), plt.scatter(), or plt.bar(). This allows you to overlay different data series or visualizations on the same plot, facilitating comparison and analysis.

3. Customization and Styling

Labels and titles: Matplotlib provides functions to add labels and titles to your plots. You can use plt.xlabel() and plt.ylabel() to set the labels for the x-axis and y-axis, respectively, and plt.title() to add a title to the plot. These labels help in clearly communicating the contents of the visualization.

Legends: When you have multiple data series or categories in a plot, adding a legend helps in distinguishing between them. Matplotlib's plt.legend() function allows you to create a legend that maps the plot elements to their corresponding labels.

Colors and styles: Matplotlib offers a wide range of color maps and styles to customize the appearance of your plots. You can set the colors of lines, markers, and plot elements using color names, hexadecimal codes, or color maps. Additionally, you can control line styles, marker styles, and other visual properties to enhance the aesthetics of your visualizations.

5.4.2 Seaborn

Seaborn is a statistical data visualization library built on top of Matplotlib. It provides a high-level interface for creating attractive and informative statistical graphics. Seaborn simplifies the process of creating complex visualizations by providing default styles and color palettes that are aesthetically pleasing and effective in conveying data insights.

1. Statistical Plots

Distribution plots: Seaborn offers several functions for visualizing the distribution of a variable, such as sns.histplot() for creating histograms, sns.kdeplot() for kernel density estimation plots, and sns.rugplot() for adding rug marks to visualize individual data points.

Categorical plots: Seaborn provides functions for visualizing categorical data, such as sns.countplot() for displaying the count of observations in each category, sns.barplot() for comparing the mean or median of a variable across categories, and sns.boxplot() for showing the distribution of a variable within categories using box plots.

Relationship plots: Seaborn offers functions to visualize the relationship between variables, such as sns.scatterplot() for creating scatter plots, sns.lineplot() for line plots, and sns.regplot() for adding regression lines to scatter plots.

2. Multi-Plot Grids

Facet grids: Seaborn's sns.FacetGrid allows you to create a grid of subplots based on one or more categorical variables. This is useful when you want to visualize the relationship between variables across different subsets of the data. You can specify the row and column variables, and Seaborn will create a grid of plots accordingly.

Pair plots: The sns.pairplot() function creates a matrix of scatter plots showing the pairwise relationships between variables in a dataset. It provides a quick way to visualize the correlations and distributions of multiple variables simultaneously.

3. Styling and Aesthetics

Seaborn themes: Seaborn offers a set of built-in themes that control the overall look and feel of the plots. You can use functions like sns.set_style() to set the plot style (e.g., "darkgrid", "whitegrid", "ticks") and sns.set_context() to set the context (e.g., "paper", "notebook", "talk") which adjusts the scaling of plot elements.

Color palettes: Seaborn provides a variety of color palettes that are visually appealing and suitable for different types of data. You can use functions like sns.color_palette() to create and customize color palettes based on different schemes (e.g., "viridis", "coolwarm", "hls") or manually specify your own colors.

When applying Matplotlib and Seaborn to healthcare data visualization, consider the following examples:

a. Patient Demographics:

Use Seaborn's sns.countplot() to display the distribution of patients across different age groups, gender categories, or ethnicities.

Create a bar plot using Matplotlib's plt.bar() to compare the prevalence of specific medical conditions across different patient groups.

b. Clinical Measurements:

Utilize Seaborn's sns.histplot() or sns.kdeplot() to visualize the distribution of clinical measurements, such as blood pressure, glucose levels, or BMI, across the patient population.

Create a scatter plot using Matplotlib's plt.scatter() to explore the relationship between two clinical variables, such as cholesterol levels and age.

c. Treatment Outcomes:

Use Seaborn's sns.barplot() to compare the effectiveness of different treatment options based on patient outcomes or recovery rates.

Create a line plot using Matplotlib's plt.plot() to track the progression of a patient's vital signs or disease markers over time.

d. Longitudinal Analysis:

Utilize Seaborn's sns.lineplot() to visualize the changes in patient metrics or biomarkers over an extended period, such as the progression of a chronic condition.

Create subplots using Matplotlib's plt.subplots() to display multiple patient trajectories or compare the longitudinal patterns across different patient subgroups.

e. Heatmaps and Correlation Matrices:

Use Seaborn's sns.heatmap() to create a heatmap visualization of correlation matrices, allowing you to identify relationships and patterns among multiple clinical variables.

Customize the heatmap with appropriate color schemes, labels, and annotations to enhance readability and interpretability.

When creating visualizations of healthcare data, it's crucial to consider the audience and purpose of the visualizations. Tailor your plots to effectively communicate the key insights and trends to healthcare professionals, researchers, or patients. Use clear labels, informative titles, and appropriate color schemes to ensure that the visualizations are easily understandable and visually appealing.

Additionally, be mindful of data privacy and confidentiality when visualizing healthcare data. Ensure that any visualizations you create do not disclose sensitive patient information or violate privacy regulations. Anonymize or aggregate data as necessary to protect patient privacy while still conveying meaningful insights.

Matplotlib and Seaborn provide a powerful toolkit for creating a wide range of visualizations suitable for healthcare data analysis. One can explore and communicate patterns, relationships, and trends in healthcare datasets, enabling data-driven decision-making and facilitating effective communication among healthcare stakeholders by using these libraries.

5.5 Case Study 1: Analyzing Patient Data
5.5.1 Objective

In this case study, we will explore how to analyze patient data using Python libraries such as NumPy, Pandas, Matplotlib, and Seaborn. We will load a dataset containing patient information, perform data manipulation and analysis, and create visualizations to gain insights into patient demographics, clinical measurements, and treatment outcomes.

5.5.2 Dataset

We will use a fictional dataset called "patient_data.csv" which contains the following columns:

Patient ID: Unique identifier for each patient

Age: Age of the patient

Gender: Gender of the patient (Male/Female)

BMI: Body Mass Index of the patient

Glucose: Blood glucose level of the patient

Blood Pressure: Blood pressure of the patient (Systolic/Diastolic)

Cholesterol: Cholesterol level of the patient

Smoking: Smoking status of the patient (Yes/No)

Alcohol Intake: Alcohol intake status of the patient (Yes/No)

Physical Activity: Physical activity level of the patient (Low/Moderate/High)

Cardiovascular Disease: Presence of cardiovascular disease (Yes/No)

Steps:

Data Loading

- Use Pandas' pd.read_csv() function to load the "patient_data.csv" file into a DataFrame.
- Explore the initial structure of the DataFrame using functions like head(), info(), and describe() to get an overview of the data.

Data Preprocessing

- Check for missing values in the dataset using isnull().sum() and handle them appropriately (e.g., dropping rows or filling with suitable values).
- Convert categorical variables (e.g., Gender, Smoking, Alcohol Intake) into numerical representations using techniques like label encoding or one-hot encoding.

Data Analysis

- Analyze the distribution of age, BMI, glucose, blood pressure, and cholesterol using Pandas' describe() function and Matplotlib's histogram plots.
- Explore the relationship between different variables, such as age and BMI, using Seaborn's scatter plots or pair plots.
- Investigate the prevalence of cardiovascular disease across different patient groups using Seaborn's bar plots or Matplotlib's pie charts.

Data Visualization

- Create a histogram plot using Matplotlib to visualize the distribution of age in the patient population.
- Use Seaborn's violin plot or box plot to compare the distribution of BMI across different physical activity levels.
- Generate a heatmap using Seaborn to visualize the correlation matrix between numerical variables like age, BMI, glucose, blood pressure, and cholesterol.
- Create a stacked bar plot using Matplotlib to display the

proportion of patients with and without cardiovascular disease across different age groups.

Insights and Conclusions
- Interpret the results of the data analysis and visualizations to derive meaningful insights about the patient population.
- Identify any patterns or relationships between variables that may be relevant for understanding patient health and guiding treatment decisions.
- Discuss the limitations of the analysis and potential areas for further investigation or data collection.

5.6 Case Study 2: Analyzing Hospital Readmission Rates

5.6.1 Objective

In this case study, we will analyze hospital readmission rates using Python libraries to identify factors that contribute to patient readmissions and develop strategies to reduce readmission rates. We will load a dataset containing patient information and readmission details, perform data manipulation and analysis, and create visualizations to gain insights into readmission patterns and associated risk factors.

5.6.2 Dataset

We will use a fictional dataset called "hospital_readmissions.csv" which contains the following columns:

Patient ID: Unique identifier for each patient

Age: Age of the patient

Gender: Gender of the patient (Male/Female)

Diagnosis: Primary diagnosis of the patient

Length of Stay: Number of days the patient stayed in the hospital during the initial admission

Comorbidities: Number of comorbidities (co-existing medical conditions) of the patient

Discharge Disposition: Discharge disposition of the patient (e.g., Home, Skilled Nursing Facility)

Readmission: Whether the patient was readmitted within 30 days (Yes/No)

5.6.3 Steps

Data Loading

Use Pandas' pd.read_csv() function to load the "hospital_readmissions.csv" file into a DataFrame.

Explore the initial structure of the DataFrame using functions like head(), info(), and describe() to get an overview of the data.

Data Preprocessing:

- Check for missing values in the dataset using isnull().sum() and handle them appropriately (e.g., dropping rows or filling with suitable values).
- Convert categorical variables (e.g., Gender, Diagnosis, Discharge Disposition) into numerical representations using techniques like label encoding or one-hot encoding.

5.6.4 Data Analysis

- Analyze the distribution of age, length of stay, and comorbidities using Pandas' describe() function and Matplotlib's histogram plots.
- Explore the relationship between different variables, such as age and readmission, using Seaborn's violin plots or box plots.
- Investigate the readmission rates across different diagnosis groups or discharge dispositions using Seaborn's bar plots or Matplotlib's stacked bar plots.

5.6.5 Data Visualization

- Create a bar plot using Matplotlib to visualize the readmission rates for different age groups.
- Use Seaborn's swarm plot or strip plot to compare the length of stay between readmitted and non-readmitted patients.
- Generate a heatmap using Seaborn to visualize the

correlation matrix between numerical variables like age, length of stay, and comorbidities.

- Create a grouped bar plot using Matplotlib to display the readmission rates across different discharge dispositions and diagnosis groups.

5.6.6 Insights and Conclusions

- Interpret the results of the data analysis and visualizations to identify factors that contribute to hospital readmissions.

- Discuss potential strategies or interventions that could be implemented to reduce readmission rates based on the identified risk factors.

- Highlight any limitations of the analysis and suggest areas for further research or data collection to improve readmission prediction and prevention.

5.7 Case Study 3: Analyzing Clinical Trial Data

5.7.1 Objective

In this case study, we will analyze clinical trial data using Python libraries to assess the efficacy and safety of a new drug treatment. We will load a dataset containing patient information and trial outcomes, perform data manipulation and analysis, and create visualizations to evaluate the treatment effects and identify any adverse events.

5.7.2 Dataset

We will use a fictional dataset called "clinical_trial_data.csv" which contains the following columns:

Patient ID: Unique identifier for each patient

Age: Age of the patient

Gender: Gender of the patient (Male/Female)

Treatment Group: Treatment group assigned to the patient (Treatment/Placebo)

Baseline Measure: Baseline measurement of the primary outcome variable

Week 4 Measure: Measurement of the primary outcome variable at Week 4

Week 8 Measure: Measurement of the primary outcome variable at Week 8

Week 12 Measure: Measurement of the primary outcome variable at Week 12

Adverse Event: Presence of any adverse event during the trial (Yes/No)

Steps

1. Data Loading

Use Pandas' pd.read_csv() function to load the "clinical_trial_data.csv" file into a DataFrame.

Explore the initial structure of the DataFrame using functions like head(), info(), and describe() to get an overview of the data.

2. Data Preprocessing

Check for missing values in the dataset using isnull().sum() and handle them appropriately (e.g., dropping rows or filling with suitable values).

Convert categorical variables (e.g., Gender, Treatment Group, Adverse Event) into numerical representations using techniques like label encoding or one-hot encoding.

3. Data Analysis

Analyze the distribution of age and baseline measurements using Pandas' describe() function and Matplotlib's histogram plots.

Explore the change in the primary outcome variable over time (Week 4, Week 8, Week 12) for both treatment and placebo groups using Seaborn's line plots or Matplotlib's scatter plots.

Investigate the occurrence of adverse events across different age groups or gender using Seaborn's bar plots or Matplotlib's stacked bar plots.

4. Data Visualization

Create a line plot using Matplotlib to visualize the change in the primary outcome variable over time for both treatment and placebo groups.

Use Seaborn's box plots or violin plots to compare the distribution of the primary outcome variable between treatment and placebo groups at different time points.

Generate a bar plot using Matplotlib to display the proportion of patients experiencing adverse events in each treatment group.

Create a scatter plot using Seaborn to explore the relationship between age and the change in the primary outcome variable from baseline to Week 12.

5. Insights and Conclusions

Interpret the results of the data analysis and visualizations to assess the efficacy of the new drug treatment compared to the placebo.

Evaluate any significant differences in the primary outcome variable between the treatment and placebo groups at different time points.

Discuss the prevalence of adverse events and any potential associations with patient characteristics like age or gender.

Provide recommendations for further clinical trials or considerations for the use of the new drug treatment based on the analysis findings

6 MACHINE LEARNING APPLICATIONS IN HEALTHCARE WITH PYTHON

6.1 Introduction to Machine Learning

Machine learning is a branch of artificial intelligence that focuses on developing algorithms and models that enable computers to learn and make predictions or decisions without being explicitly programmed. In the context of healthcare, machine learning has the potential to revolutionize the way we diagnose diseases, develop personalized treatment plans, and improve patient outcomes. Machine learning algorithms can uncover hidden patterns by utilizing the vast amounts of medical data available, identify risk factors, and assist healthcare professionals in making data-driven decisions.

6.2 Types of Machine Learning
6.2.1 Supervised Learning

In supervised learning, the algorithm learns from labeled data, where both the input features and corresponding output labels are provided. The goal is to learn a mapping function that can predict the output for new, unseen input data. Common supervised learning algorithms include linear regression, logistic regression, decision trees, and support vector machines.

6.2.2 Unsupervised Learning

Unsupervised learning deals with unlabeled data, where only the input features are available, and the algorithm aims to discover inherent patterns or structures in the data. Clustering and dimensionality reduction are common unsupervised learning techniques. Examples include k-means clustering, hierarchical clustering, and principal component analysis.

6.2.3 Semi-Supervised Learning

Semi-supervised learning lies between supervised and unsupervised learning, where a small portion of the data is labeled, and the majority is unlabeled. The algorithm learns from both labeled and unlabeled data to improve its performance. Semi-supervised learning is particularly useful when labeled data is scarce or expensive to obtain.

6.2.4 Reinforcement Learning

Reinforcement learning involves an agent that learns to make decisions by interacting with an environment. The agent receives rewards or penalties based on its actions and aims to maximize the cumulative reward over time. Reinforcement learning is commonly used in robotics, gaming, and decision-making systems.

6.3 Machine Learning Process
6.3.1 Data Collection

The first step in the machine learning process is to collect relevant data. In healthcare, this may involve gathering patient records, medical images, sensor data, or genomic information. It's essential to ensure that the data is representative, diverse, and of high quality.

6.3.2 Data Preprocessing

Raw data often requires preprocessing before it can be used for machine learning. This step involves cleaning the data, handling missing values, outliers, and inconsistencies. Data normalization or standardization may be applied to ensure that all features are on a similar scale. Feature selection or engineering techniques can be used to extract relevant features from the data.

6.3.3 Model Selection

Based on the nature of the problem and the available data, an appropriate machine learning algorithm is selected. The choice of algorithm depends on factors such as the type of task (classification, regression, clustering), the size and complexity of the data, and the desired interpretability of the model.

6.3.4 Model Training

The selected algorithm is trained on a portion of the preprocessed data, known as the training set. During training, the model learns the underlying patterns and relationships in the data by adjusting its internal parameters. The goal is to minimize the difference between the model's predictions and the actual outcomes.

6.3.5 Model Evaluation

After training, the model's performance is evaluated on a separate portion of the data, called the validation or test set. Evaluation metrics such as accuracy, precision, recall, F1-score, or mean squared error are used to assess the model's predictive power. Cross-validation techniques can be employed to obtain more reliable performance estimates.

6.3.6 Model Deployment

Once the model achieves satisfactory performance, it can be deployed in a production environment to make predictions on new, unseen data. The model's predictions can be integrated into clinical decision support systems, personalized treatment recommendations, or early warning systems for disease detection

6.4 Machine Learning Libraries in Python

Scikit-learn

Scikit-learn is a popular machine learning library in Python that provides a wide range of supervised and unsupervised learning algorithms. It offers a consistent interface for model training, evaluation, and prediction, making it easy to experiment with different algorithms and compare their performance.

TensorFlow

TensorFlow is an open-source library developed by

Google for machine learning and deep learning. It provides a flexible ecosystem for building and deploying machine learning models, with a focus on neural networks and deep learning architectures. TensorFlow is widely used for tasks such as image classification, natural language processing, and time series forecasting.

PyTorch

PyTorch is an open-source machine learning library developed by Facebook. It provides a dynamic computational graph and supports both deep learning and traditional machine learning algorithms. PyTorch is known for its ease of use, flexibility, and strong support for research and experimentation.

XGBoost

XGBoost (Extreme Gradient Boosting) is a powerful library for gradient boosting, which is an ensemble learning technique that combines multiple weak learners to create a strong predictive model. XGBoost is known for its excellent performance, scalability, and ability to handle large-scale datasets efficiently.

Keras

Keras is a high-level neural networks library that can run on top of TensorFlow, Theano, or CNTK. It provides a user-friendly interface for building and training deep learning models, making it accessible to beginners and practitioners alike. Keras supports various types of neural networks, including convolutional neural networks (CNNs) and recurrent neural networks (RNNs).

6.5 Applications of Machine Learning in Healthcare

Disease Diagnosis

Machine learning algorithms can assist in the early detection and diagnosis of diseases by analyzing medical images, patient records, or biomarkers. For example, deep learning models can be trained to detect abnormalities in X-rays, CT scans, or MRI images, aiding radiologists in identifying potential health issues.

Risk Prediction

Machine learning models can predict the likelihood of a patient developing certain diseases or experiencing adverse events based on their clinical history, lifestyle factors, and genetic information. These predictions can help healthcare providers take proactive measures and personalize preventive care strategies.

Treatment Optimization

Machine learning can be used to optimize treatment plans by analyzing patient data, treatment outcomes, and side effects. Models can suggest personalized treatment regimens by identifying patterns and correlations that maximize the chances of success while minimizing potential risks.

Drug Discovery

Machine learning techniques can accelerate the drug discovery process by predicting the potential efficacy and safety of new drug compounds., models can identify promising drug candidates and guide the design of targeted therapies by analyzing large datasets of molecular structures and their properties.

Patient Monitoring

Machine learning algorithms can analyze real-time data from wearable devices, sensors, or electronic health records to monitor patients' health status remotely. This enables early detection of deteriorating conditions, timely interventions, and improved patient outcomes, especially for chronic diseases or post-operative care.

Clinical Decision Support

Machine learning models can provide data-driven insights and recommendations to healthcare professionals, assisting them in making informed decisions. Healthcare providers can improve diagnostic accuracy, treatment selection, and patient management by integrating machine learning predictions with clinical expertise.

6.6 Ethical Considerations and Challenges

Data Privacy and Security

Healthcare data is highly sensitive and subject to strict privacy regulations. When applying machine learning to healthcare, it is crucial to ensure that patient data is securely stored, anonymized, and used in compliance with ethical guidelines and legal requirements.

Bias and Fairness

Machine learning models can inadvertently inherit biases present in the training data, leading to discriminatory or unfair predictions. It is essential to carefully curate diverse and representative datasets and employ techniques to mitigate bias and ensure fairness in model predictions.

Interpretability and Transparency

Many machine learning models, especially deep learning algorithms, are often considered "black boxes" due to their complex internal workings. Ensuring interpretability and transparency of machine learning models is crucial in healthcare to build trust, enable clinical validation, and facilitate regulatory approval.

Regulatory and Legal Challenges

The application of machine learning in healthcare is subject to regulatory and legal frameworks. Ensuring compliance with medical device regulations, obtaining necessary approvals, and addressing liability concerns are important considerations when deploying machine learning systems in clinical settings

6.7 Scikit-learn for Predictive Modeling

Scikit-learn is a powerful and widely used machine learning library in Python. It provides a comprehensive set of tools for building predictive models, including various supervised and unsupervised learning algorithms.

In this section, we will explore how to use scikit-learn for predictive modeling in healthcare.

6.7.1 Installation and Setup

To get started with scikit-learn, you need to have Python installed on your system. You can install scikit-learn using pip, the Python package installer, by running the following command:

pip install scikit-learn

Once installed, you can import the necessary modules from scikit-learn in your Python script or Jupyter Notebook:

```
From sklearn import datasets, model_selection, metrics
from sklearn.linear_model import LogisticRegression
from sklearn.tree import DecisionTreeClassifier
from sklearn.ensemble import RandomForestClassifier
```

6.7.2 Loading and Preprocessing Data

Scikit-learn provides built-in datasets that can be used for learning and experimentation. For example, you can load the breast cancer dataset using the following code:

```
from sklearn.datasets import load_breast_cancer
data = load_breast_cancer()
X, y = data.data, data.target
```

In real-world scenarios, you would typically load your own healthcare dataset from a file or database. Scikit-learn supports various data formats, such as CSV, Excel, or SQL databases.

Before training a model, you may need to preprocess the data. Scikit-learn offers a range of preprocessing techniques, including scaling, normalization, encoding categorical variables, and handling missing values. For example, to scale the features using StandardScaler:

```
from sklearn.preprocessing import StandardScaler
scaler = StandardScaler()
X_scaled = scaler.fit_transform(X)
```

6.7.3. Model Selection and Training

Scikit-learn provides a wide range of supervised

learning algorithms for predictive modeling. Some commonly used algorithms include logistic regression, decision trees, random forests, support vector machines, and naive Bayes.

To train a model, you first create an instance of the desired algorithm and then fit it to the training data. For example, to train a logistic regression model:

```
from sklearn.linear_model import LogisticRegression
model = LogisticRegression()
model.fit(X_train, y_train)
Scikit-learn also provides a model selection module that allows
you to perform cross-validation and hyperparameter tuning. For
example, to perform 5-fold cross-validation:
from sklearn.model_selection import cross_val_score
scores = cross_val_score(model, X, y, cv=5)
print("Cross-validation scores:", scores)
```

6.7.4 Model Evaluation

After training a model, it's crucial to evaluate its performance on unseen data. Scikit-learn provides various evaluation metrics for classification and regression tasks.

For classification, common metrics include accuracy, precision, recall, F1-score, and area under the ROC curve (AUC-ROC). For example, to calculate the accuracy of a model:

```
from sklearn.metrics import accuracy_score
y_pred = model.predict(X_test)
accuracy = accuracy_score(y_test, y_pred)
print("Accuracy:", accuracy)
```

For regression, metrics such as mean squared error (MSE), mean absolute error (MAE), and R-squared are commonly used. For example, to calculate the mean squared error:

```
from sklearn.metrics import mean_squared_error
y_pred = model.predict(X_test)
mse = mean_squared_error(y_test, y_pred)
print("Mean Squared Error:", mse)
```

6.7.5 Model Interpretation and Feature Importance

Understanding the factors that influence the model's predictions is essential in healthcare applications. Scikit-learn provides methods to interpret models and assess feature importance.

For linear models like logistic regression, you can access the model coefficients to understand the impact of each feature on the prediction. For example:

```
coefficients = model.coef_
print("Model coefficients:", coefficients)
```

Tree-based models like decision trees and random forests allow you to compute feature importances, indicating the relative contribution of each feature to the model's predictions. For example:

```
importances = model.feature_importances_
print("Feature importances:", importances)
```

6.7.6. Deploying and Updating Models

Once a model is trained and evaluated, it can be deployed in a production environment to make predictions on new, unseen data. Scikit-learn models can be easily serialized and saved to disk using the joblib library:

```
import joblib
joblib.dump(model, 'model.pkl')
```

To load a saved model and make predictions:

```
loaded_model = joblib.load('model.pkl')
predictions = loaded_model.predict(new_data)
```

As new data becomes available, it's important to continuously update and retrain the models to adapt to changing patterns and maintain high performance. Scikit-learn's model persistence capabilities make it convenient to update models incrementally.

Scikit-learn provides a comprehensive and user-friendly framework for building predictive models in healthcare. Its extensive collection of algorithms, preprocessing techniques, and evaluation metrics makes it a valuable tool for healthcare data scientists and researchers.

Here are a few examples of how scikit-learn can be applied in healthcare predictive modeling:

Disease Prediction: Using logistic regression or decision trees to predict the likelihood of a patient developing a specific disease based on their clinical features and risk factors.

Readmission Risk Assessment: Building a random forest model to predict the probability of a patient being readmitted to the hospital within a certain timeframe based on their demographic, clinical, and historical data.

Survival Analysis: Utilizing scikit-learn's survival analysis module to model and predict patient survival probabilities based on various prognostic factors.

Treatment Response Prediction: Applying support vector machines or gradient boosting algorithms to predict a patient's response to a specific treatment based on their genetic profile, medical history, and clinical measurements.

6.8 Case Study 1: Predicting Patient Readmission

Objective

The goal of this case study is to develop a predictive model using scikit-learn to identify patients who are at high risk of being readmitted to the hospital within 30 days of discharge. Healthcare providers can allocate resources and interventions to prevent unnecessary readmissions and improve patient outcomes by accurately predicting readmission risk.

Dataset

We will use a publicly available dataset called the "Diabetes 130-US hospitals for years 1999-2008" dataset. This dataset contains information about hospital admissions of patients with diabetes, including demographic data, diagnostic codes, medication information, and readmission status.

Steps

1. Data Preprocessing:

a. Load the dataset and perform necessary data cleaning and preprocessing steps.

b. Handle missing values, encode categorical variables, and scale numerical features.

c. Split the dataset into training and testing sets.

2. Feature Selection
a. Identify relevant features that may contribute to readmission risk, such as age, gender, comorbidities, length of stay, and medication information.
b. Use feature selection techniques like correlation analysis or recursive feature elimination to select the most informative features.

3. Model Training
a. Choose an appropriate algorithm for the prediction task, such as logistic regression, decision trees, or random forests.
b. Train the selected model on the training data using scikit-learn's fit() method.
c. Optimize the model's hyperparameters using techniques like grid search or randomized search.

4. Model Evaluation
a. Evaluate the trained model's performance on the testing data using metrics such as accuracy, precision, recall, and F1-score.
b. Analyze the confusion matrix to assess the model's ability to correctly identify readmitted and non-readmitted patients.
c. Consider using cross-validation to obtain more robust performance estimates.

5. Model Interpretation
a. Examine the model's coefficients or feature importances to understand the relative contribution of each feature to the readmission prediction.
b. Visualize the model's decision boundaries or feature relationships using techniques like decision tree visualization or partial dependence plots.

6. Model Deployment

a. Save the trained model using scikit-learn's joblib or pickle modules.

b. Integrate the model into a clinical decision support system or a web application for real-time readmission risk prediction.

c. Continuously monitor and update the model as new data becomes available to ensure its performance and reliability.

6.9 Case Study 2: Predicting Breast Cancer Diagnosis

Objective

The goal of this case study is to develop a predictive model using scikit-learn to classify breast cancer tumors as benign or malignant based on various diagnostic measurements. Accurate prediction of breast cancer diagnosis can assist healthcare professionals in making informed decisions regarding patient management and treatment planning.

Dataset

We will use the "Breast Cancer Wisconsin (Diagnostic)" dataset, which contains features computed from digitized images of fine needle aspirate (FNA) of breast mass. The dataset includes measurements such as radius, texture, perimeter, area, smoothness, and concavity of the cell nuclei.

Steps

1. Data Preprocessing

a. Load the dataset and perform necessary data cleaning and preprocessing steps.

b. Handle missing values, if any, and scale the features to a common range.

c. Split the dataset into training and testing sets.

2. Exploratory Data Analysis

a. Visualize the distribution of features and their relationship with the target variable (benign or malignant).

b. Identify any potential outliers or imbalanced classes that may require special handling.

3. Model Training

a. Select appropriate classification algorithms, such as logistic regression, decision trees, random forests, or support vector machines.

b. Train the chosen models on the training data using scikit-learn's fit() method.

c. Perform hyperparameter tuning using techniques like grid search or randomized search to optimize model performance.

4. Model Evaluation

a. Evaluate the trained models' performance on the testing data using metrics such as accuracy, precision, recall, and F1-score.

b. Analyze the confusion matrix to assess the models' ability to correctly classify benign and malignant tumors.

c. Employ cross-validation techniques to obtain more reliable performance estimates.

5. Model Comparison and Selection

a. Compare the performance of different models and select the best-performing model based on the evaluation metrics.

b.Consider the interpretability and computational efficiency of the models in addition to their predictive performance.

6. Model Interpretation

a. Examine the selected model's coefficients or feature importances to identify the most influential features in predicting breast cancer diagnosis.

b. Visualize the model's decision boundaries or feature relationships using techniques like decision tree visualization or principal component analysis (PCA).

7. Model Deployment and Integration

a. Save the trained model using scikit-learn's joblib or pickle modules.

b. Integrate the model into a clinical decision support system or a web application for real-time breast cancer diagnosis prediction.

c. Ensure proper validation and regulatory compliance before deploying the model in a production environment.

6.10 Case Study 3: Predicting Patient Mortality Risk

Objective

The goal of this case study is to develop a predictive model using scikit-learn to assess the mortality risk of patients in an intensive care unit (ICU) based on various clinical parameters and demographic information. Accurate prediction of mortality risk can assist healthcare providers in making informed decisions regarding treatment intensification, resource allocation, and end-of-life care planning.

Dataset

We will use the "MIMIC-III" (Medical Information Mart for Intensive Care) dataset, which contains de-identified health-related data associated with ICU patients. The dataset includes variables such as demographics, vital signs, laboratory tests, medications, and patient outcomes.

Steps

1. Data Preprocessing

a. Extract relevant features from the MIMIC-III dataset, such as age, gender, comorbidities, vital signs, and laboratory results.

b. Handle missing values, normalize or standardize the features, and encode categorical variables.

c. Define the target variable as the mortality status (deceased or survived) of patients.

2.Feature Engineering

a. Create new features based on domain knowledge or clinical expertise, such as the Acute Physiology and Chronic Health Evaluation (APACHE) score or the Sequential Organ Failure Assessment (SOFA) score.

b. Utilize temporal information by aggregating or summarizing time-series data, such as the average heart rate over a specific period.

3. Model Training

a. Select appropriate algorithms for mortality risk prediction, such as logistic regression, gradient boosting machines, or neural networks.

b. Train the chosen models on the preprocessed dataset using scikit-learn's fit() method.

c. Perform hyperparameter tuning using techniques like grid search or Bayesian optimization to optimize model performance.

4. Model Evaluation

a. Evaluate the trained models' performance using metrics such as area under the receiver operating characteristic curve (AUC-ROC), precision-recall curve, and calibration plots.

b. Assess the models' performance across different subgroups or time horizons to ensure robustness and generalizability.

c. Employ techniques like nested cross-validation to obtain unbiased performance estimates.

5. Model Interpretation

a. Analyze the selected model's coefficients or feature importances to identify the most influential predictors of mortality risk.

b. Visualize the model's decision boundaries or risk scores using techniques like partial dependence plots or Shapley additive explanations (SHAP).

6. Model Validation and Deployment

a. Validate the model's performance on an independent test set or an external validation cohort to assess its generalizability.

b. Integrate the trained model into a clinical decision support system or a web-based tool for real-time mortality risk assessment.

c. Establish proper monitoring and updating procedures to ensure the model's performance remains stable over time.

7. Ethical Considerations

a. Address ethical considerations related to the use of predictive models in critical care settings, such as ensuring fairness, transparency, and patient privacy.

b. Engage with healthcare professionals and stakeholders to discuss the implications and limitations of the mortality risk prediction model.

b. Ensure that the model's predictions are used as a supportive tool and do not replace clinical judgment or patient-centered decision-making.

7 NATURAL LANGUAGE PROCESSING FOR ELECTRONIC HEALTH RECORDS WITH PYTHON

7.1 Introduction to Natural Language Processing

Natural Language Processing (NLP) is a branch of artificial intelligence that focuses on the interaction between computers and human language. It involves the development of algorithms and models that enable computers to understand, interpret, and generate human language in a meaningful way. NLP has numerous applications in healthcare, particularly in the analysis and extraction of information from electronic health records (EHRs).

7.2 Importance of NLP in Healthcare

Electronic Health Records (EHRs) contain a wealth of information, including structured data (e.g., patient demographics, diagnosis codes) and unstructured data (e.g., clinical notes, discharge summaries).

Unstructured data in EHRs often contains valuable insights, such as patient symptoms, medical history, treatment plans, and outcomes. However, manually reviewing and extracting information from unstructured text is time-consuming and inefficient.

NLP techniques can automate the process of extracting relevant information from unstructured EHR data, enabling healthcare professionals to access key insights quickly and efficiently.

NLP can assist in various healthcare applications, such as clinical decision support, patient cohort identification, adverse event detection, and population health management.

7.3 Key Concepts in NLP

Tokenization: Tokenization is the process of breaking down text into smaller units called tokens. Tokens can be individual words, phrases, or subwords. Tokenization is a fundamental step in NLP, as it allows for further processing and analysis of the text.

Part-of-Speech (POS) Tagging: POS tagging involves assigning grammatical tags to each token in a text, such as noun, verb, adjective, or adverb. POS tagging helps in understanding the syntactic structure of the text and can be useful for tasks like named entity recognition and information extraction.

Named Entity Recognition (NER): NER is the process of identifying and classifying named entities in text, such as person names, organizations, locations, medical concepts, and medications. NER is particularly relevant in healthcare NLP, as it enables the extraction of key medical entities from EHRs.

Syntactic Parsing: Syntactic parsing involves analyzing the grammatical structure of a sentence and identifying the relationships between words. It helps in understanding the dependencies and hierarchical structure of the text, which can be useful for tasks like relation extraction and sentiment analysis.

Text Classification: Text classification is the task of assigning predefined categories or labels to a given text based on its content. In healthcare, text classification can be used to categorize clinical notes into different types (e.g., discharge summary, progress note) or to identify the presence of certain medical conditions or symptoms.

7.4 NLP Libraries in Python

Natural Language Toolkit (NLTK): NLTK is a popular open-source library for NLP in Python. It provides a wide range of tools and resources for tasks like tokenization, POS tagging, named entity recognition, and text classification. NLTK also includes various corpora and pre-trained models that can be used for NLP tasks.

spaCy: spaCy is a powerful and efficient NLP library in Python. It offers a streamlined API for common NLP tasks, such as tokenization, POS tagging, named entity recognition, and dependency parsing. spaCy is known for its speed and performance, making it suitable for processing large volumes of text data.

Gensim: Gensim is a library for topic modeling and document similarity retrieval. It provides implementations of popular algorithms like Latent Dirichlet Allocation (LDA) and Word2Vec, which can be used for tasks like document clustering, text summarization, and semantic similarity analysis.

Scikit-learn: Scikit-learn is a machine learning library in Python that also offers functionality for text preprocessing and feature extraction. It provides tools for text tokenization, vectorization (e.g., bag-of-words, TF-IDF), and text classification using various algorithms like Naive Bayes, Support Vector Machines, and Random Forests.

7.5 Preprocessing EHR Data

Data Cleaning: EHR data often contains noise, such as typographical errors, abbreviations, and inconsistent formatting. Data cleaning involves identifying and correcting these issues to ensure the quality and consistency of the text data.

Handling Abbreviations and Acronyms: Medical text frequently uses abbreviations and acronyms, which can be challenging for NLP algorithms to understand. Developing a comprehensive dictionary of medical abbreviations and their expansions is crucial for accurate text processing.

Negation Handling: Negation is common in clinical notes, where the absence or negation of a condition or symptom is mentioned (e.g., "patient denies chest pain"). Identifying and handling negation is important to avoid misinterpreting the presence of medical concepts.

Stopword Removal: Stopwords are common words that often carry little meaning in the context of NLP, such as "a," "an," "the," and "of." Removing stopwords can help reduce the dimensionality of the text data and focus on more informative words.

Stemming and Lemmatization: Stemming and lemmatization are techniques used to normalize words to their base or dictionary form. Stemming reduces words to their root form by removing suffixes, while lemmatization considers the context and converts words to their base lemma. These techniques can help group related words and reduce the vocabulary size.

7.6 Applications of NLP in EHR Analysis

NLP can be used to identify and extract clinical entities from EHRs, such as diseases, symptoms, medications, and procedures. This information can be used for tasks like patient phenotyping, cohort selection, and clinical trial recruitment.

Relation extraction helps in identifying and extracting relationships between clinical entities in EHRs. For example, extracting the relationship between a medication and its dosage, or between a symptom and its associated disease. Relation extraction can provide insights into treatment patterns, adverse events, and disease progression.

Sentiment analysis in NLP aims to determine the sentiment or opinion expressed in a given text. In the context of EHRs, sentiment analysis can be used to identify patient satisfaction, treatment adherence, or the emotional state of patients based on their clinical notes.

EHRs often contain lengthy and complex clinical narratives. Text summarization techniques in NLP can be applied to generate concise summaries of patient records, highlighting key information and reducing information overload for healthcare professionals.

NLP can assist in automatically assigning International Classification of Diseases (ICD) codes to clinical notes., NLP can streamline the coding process and improve coding accuracy by extracting relevant medical concepts and mapping them to appropriate ICD codes.

7.7 Challenges

EHRs contain sensitive patient information, and ensuring data privacy and security is paramount when applying NLP techniques. Proper de-identification and anonymization of patient data should be performed to comply with privacy regulations and protect patient confidentiality.

Medical language often includes complex terminology, acronyms, and domain-specific expressions. Developing NLP models that can effectively handle and understand medical language requires domain expertise and the use of specialized medical vocabularies and ontologies.

Clinical notes often contain contextual information that is crucial for accurate interpretation. NLP models need to consider the context and dependencies within the text to avoid misinterpretations and capture the intended meaning accurately.

Medical text can be ambiguous and contain expressions of uncertainty, such as "possible," "likely," or "suggestive of." NLP models should be designed to handle and represent uncertainty to provide a more nuanced understanding of the clinical information.

Evaluating the performance of NLP models in healthcare is challenging due to the lack of large-scale annotated datasets and the complexity of medical language. Collaboration with healthcare experts is essential for validating the outputs of NLP models and ensuring their clinical relevance and accuracy.

Natural Language Processing holds immense potential for unlocking the value of unstructured data in electronic health records., healthcare organizations can extract meaningful insights, automate clinical processes, and support data-driven decision-making by utilizing NLP techniques and Python libraries.

However, the successful application of NLP in healthcare requires a multidisciplinary approach, combining expertise in computer science, linguistics, and healthcare. It is essential to address the challenges related to data privacy, domain-specific language, and model validation to ensure the reliability and trustworthiness of NLP-based solutions.

7.8 NLTK and spaCy for Text Processing

NLTK (Natural Language Toolkit) and spaCy are two popular Python libraries for natural language processing (NLP). Both libraries provide a wide range of tools and functionalities for processing and analyzing text data. In this section, we will explore the key features and capabilities of NLTK and spaCy and demonstrate their usage for text processing tasks in the context of electronic health records (EHRs).

7.8.1 NLTK (Natural Language Toolkit)

NLTK is a comprehensive Python library for NLP, offering a diverse set of tools for text processing, linguistic analysis, and machine learning. It provides a user-friendly interface and a wide range of built-in corpora and pre-trained models for various NLP tasks.

Key features of NLTK include tokenization, part-of-speech (POS) tagging, named entity recognition (NER), sentiment analysis, and text classification.

Example: Tokenization and POS Tagging with NLTK

```
import nltk
from nltk.tokenize import word_tokenize
from nltk.tag import pos_tag
text = "The patient complained of severe abdominal pain and nausea."
tokens = word_tokenize(text)
pos_tags = pos_tag(tokens)

print("Tokens:", tokens)
print("POS Tags:", pos_tags)

Output:
Tokens: ['The', 'patient', 'complained', 'of', 'severe', 'abdominal', 'pain', 'and', 'nausea', '.']
```

POS Tags: [('The', 'DT'), ('patient', 'NN'), ('complained', 'VBD'), ('of', 'IN'), ('severe', 'JJ'), ('abdominal', 'JJ'), ('pain', 'NN'), ('and', 'CC'), ('nausea', 'NN'), ('.', '.')]

NLTK provides a simple and intuitive way to tokenize text into individual words and perform POS tagging to identify the grammatical roles of each word in the sentence.

7.8.2 spaCy

spaCy is a powerful and efficient NLP library in Python, designed for production use and large-scale text processing.

It offers a streamlined API for common NLP tasks, such as tokenization, POS tagging, dependency parsing, and named entity recognition.

spaCy is known for its speed and performance, making it suitable for processing large volumes of EHR data.

It provides pre-trained statistical models for various languages and can be easily customized and extended for domain-specific tasks.

Example: Named Entity Recognition with spaCy

```
import spacy

# Load the pre-trained English model
nlp = spacy.load("en_core_web_sm")

text = "The patient, John Doe, was diagnosed with hypertension and prescribed lisinopril 10mg daily."
doc = nlp(text)

for entity in doc.ents:
    print(entity.text, entity.label_)
```

Output

John Doe PERSON

hypertension DISEASE
lisinopril 10mg DRUG

spaCy's pre-trained models can accurately identify and classify named entities in the text, such as person names, diseases, and medications, which is particularly useful for extracting relevant information from EHRs.

7.8.3 Combining NLTK and spaCy

NLTK and spaCy can be used together to leverage the strengths of both libraries for text processing tasks.

NLTK provides a wide range of tools and resources, while spaCy offers high-performance and efficient processing capabilities.

Combining NLTK and spaCy, one can benefit from NLTK's extensive collection of corpora, pre-trained models, and linguistic resources, while utilizing spaCy's fast and scalable processing pipeline.

Example: Sentiment Analysis with NLTK and spaCy

```
import nltk
from nltk.sentiment import SentimentIntensityAnalyzer
import spacy

# Load the pre-trained English model
nlp = spacy.load("en_core_web_sm")

# Initialize the sentiment analyzer from NLTK
sia = SentimentIntensityAnalyzer()

text = "The patient expressed satisfaction with the treatment and reported significant improvement in symptoms."
doc = nlp(text)

# Perform sentiment analysis on each sentence
for sent in doc.sents:
    sentiment_scores = sia.polarity_scores(sent.text)
    print("Sentence:", sent.text)
```

```
print("Sentiment Scores:", sentiment_scores)
```
Output:

Sentence: The patient expressed satisfaction with the treatment and reported significant improvement in symptoms.

Sentiment Scores: {'neg': 0.0, 'neu': 0.508, 'pos': 0.492, 'compound': 0.7003}

In this example, we use spaCy to split the text into sentences and NLTK's SentimentIntensityAnalyzer to calculate sentiment scores for each sentence. This combination allows us to analyze the sentiment expressed in different parts of the clinical note.

7.8.4. Preprocessing Techniques

Before applying NLP techniques using NLTK or spaCy, it is essential to preprocess the text data to improve the quality and consistency of the results.

Common preprocessing techniques include:

Lowercasing: Converting all text to lowercase to ensure consistency.

Tokenization: Splitting the text into individual words or tokens.

Stopword Removal: Eliminating common words that do not carry significant meaning, such as "the," "is," and "and."

Stemming and Lemmatization: Reducing words to their base or dictionary form to normalize the text.

Handling Special Characters and Numbers: Removing or handling special characters, punctuation, and numbers based on the specific requirements of the NLP task.

Example: Preprocessing with NLTK

```
import nltk
from nltk.tokenize import word_tokenize
from nltk.corpus import stopwords
from nltk.stem import PorterStemmer

text = "The patient's blood pressure was 130/80 mmHg, and the heart rate was 75 bpm."
```

```
# Lowercase the text
text = text.lower()

# Tokenize the text
tokens = word_tokenize(text)

# Remove stopwords
stop_words = set(stopwords.words("english"))
filtered_tokens = [token for token in tokens if token not in stop_words]

# Perform stemming
stemmer = PorterStemmer()
stemmed_tokens = [stemmer.stem(token) for token in filtered_tokens]

print("Original Text:", text)
print("Preprocessed Tokens:", stemmed_tokens)
```

Output:

Original Text: the patient's blood pressure was 130/80 mmhg, and the heart rate was 75 bpm.

Preprocessed Tokens: ['patient', 'blood', 'pressur', 'wa', '130/80', 'mmhg', ',', 'heart', 'rate', 'wa', '75', 'bpm', '.']

Preprocessing the text data helps in reducing noise, normalizing the text, and focusing on the relevant information for downstream NLP tasks.

7.8.5 Advanced NLP Techniques

NLTK and spaCy provide support for various advanced NLP techniques that can be applied to EHR data analysis, such as:

Topic Modeling: Discovering latent topics or themes in a collection of documents using algorithms like Latent Dirichlet Allocation (LDA) or Non-Negative Matrix Factorization (NMF).

Text Classification: Assigning predefined categories or labels to text documents based on their content, using algorithms like Naive Bayes, Support Vector Machines

(SVM), or deep learning models.

Relation Extraction: Identifying and extracting relationships between entities in the text, such as drug-drug interactions or symptom-disease associations.

Coreference Resolution: Resolving references to the same entity within and across sentences, which is crucial for understanding the context and linking related information in EHRs.

These advanced techniques can be implemented using NLTK, spaCy, and other complementary libraries like Gensim, scikit-learn, or TensorFlow, depending on the specific requirements of the NLP task

7.8.6 Case Study 1: Extracting Information from Clinical Notes

Objective:

In this case study, we aim to extract relevant medical information from unstructured clinical notes using NLP techniques. We will focus on identifying key entities such as diseases, symptoms, medications, and procedures mentioned in the clinical text.

Dataset:

We have a dataset of 1,000 de-identified clinical notes from a hospital's EHR system. The notes include various types of documents, such as admission notes, progress notes, and discharge summaries.

Approach

1. Preprocess the clinical notes:

a. Tokenize the text into individual words and sentences using NLTK or spaCy.

b. Perform text cleaning by removing special characters, numbers, and punctuation.

c. Convert the text to lowercase to ensure consistency.

d. Remove stopwords using a predefined list of common words.

2. Named Entity Recognition (NER):

a. Use spaCy's pre-trained medical NER model (e.g., "en_core_med7_lg") to identify medical entities in the clinical notes.
b. Extract entities such as diseases, symptoms, medications, and procedures.
c. Store the extracted entities along with their corresponding entity types.

3. Relation Extraction:
a. Identify and extract relationships between the extracted entities using dependency parsing and rule-based techniques.
b. Focus on extracting relations such as symptom-disease, medication-indication, and procedure-diagnosis pairs.
c. Store the extracted relations in a structured format for further analysis.

4. Evaluation and Validation:
a. Manually review a subset of the extracted entities and relations to assess their accuracy and relevance.
b. Collaborate with healthcare professionals to validate the extracted information and gather feedback for improvement.

5. Insights and Applications:
a. Analyze the extracted entities and relations to gain insights into disease prevalence, common symptoms, frequently prescribed medications, and treatment patterns.
b. Use the extracted information to support clinical decision-making, population health management, and research activities.

Results: We successfully extracted relevant medical entities and relationships from the clinical notes by applying NLP techniques using NLTK and spaCy. The extracted information provided valuable insights into patient conditions, treatment patterns, and disease management. The accuracy of the extracted entities and relations was evaluated and validated by healthcare experts, ensuring their clinical relevance.

The case study demonstrates the potential of NLP in automating the extraction of structured information from unstructured clinical text, enabling more efficient and data-driven healthcare processes.

7.8.7 Case Study 2: Sentiment Analysis of Patient Feedback

Objective

In this case study, we aim to analyze patient feedback from surveys and online reviews to understand patient satisfaction and identify areas for improvement in healthcare services.

Dataset

We have a dataset of 5,000 patient feedback comments collected from various sources, including post-visit surveys, online review platforms, and social media.

Approach

1. *Preprocess the patient feedback comments*

   a. Tokenize the text into individual words and sentences using NLTK or spaCy.

   b. Perform text cleaning by removing special characters, numbers, and punctuation.

   c. Convert the text to lowercase to ensure consistency.

   d. Remove stopwords using a predefined list of common words.

2. *Sentiment Analysis*

   a. Use NLTK's Sentiment Intensity Analyzer (SIA) to calculate sentiment scores for each feedback comment.

   b. Classify the comments into positive, negative, and neutral sentiments based on the sentiment scores.

   c. Identify the most common positive and negative

words or phrases associated with patient satisfaction.

3. Topic Modeling

a. Apply topic modeling techniques, such as Latent Dirichlet Allocation (LDA), to discover underlying topics or themes in the patient feedback comments.

b. Identify the most prevalent topics and their associated keywords to understand the main areas of concern or satisfaction for patients.

4. Visualization and Reporting

a. Create visualizations, such as sentiment distribution charts and word clouds, to present the sentiment analysis results in an intuitive manner.

b. Generate reports summarizing the key findings, including overall patient satisfaction levels, top positive and negative aspects, and identified areas for improvement.

5. Insights and Applications:

a. Use the sentiment analysis insights to identify strengths and weaknesses in healthcare service delivery and patient experience.

b. Prioritize improvement efforts based on the identified areas of concern and patient feedback.

c. Monitor sentiment trends over time to track the impact of implemented changes and interventions.

Results

We gained valuable insights into patient satisfaction and identified key areas for improvement in healthcare services by applying sentiment analysis and topic modeling techniques using NLTK and spaCy. The sentiment analysis revealed that a majority of patients had positive experiences, with specific aspects such as staff friendliness and cleanliness being highly appreciated. However, wait times and communication were identified as areas requiring attention.

The topic modeling analysis uncovered recurring themes in patient feedback, including appointment scheduling, billing processes, and quality of care. These insights provided actionable recommendations for enhancing patient experience and addressing specific pain points.

The case study showcases the power of NLP in analyzing patient feedback and deriving meaningful insights to drive improvements in healthcare delivery and patient satisfaction.

7.8.8 Case Study 3: Predicting Hospital Readmissions

Objective

In this case study, we aim to predict the likelihood of hospital readmissions based on information extracted from patients' discharge summaries using NLP techniques.

Dataset

We have a dataset of 10,000 de-identified discharge summaries along with corresponding patient demographic information and readmission labels (readmitted within 30 days or not).

Approach

1. *Preprocess the discharge summaries*

   a. *Tokenize the text into individual words and sentences using NLTK or spaCy.*

   b. *Perform text cleaning by removing special characters, numbers, and punctuation.*

   c. *Convert the text to lowercase to ensure consistency.*

   d. *Remove stopwords using a predefined list of common words.*

2. *Feature Extraction*

   a. Extract relevant features from the discharge summaries using NLP techniques:

   b. Use spaCy's pre-trained medical NER model to identify medical entities such as diseases, medications, and procedures.

   c. Apply sentiment analysis using NLTK's SIA to

capture the overall sentiment expressed in the discharge summaries.

d. Utilize topic modeling techniques like LDA to identify dominant topics or themes in the discharge summaries.

3. Combining NLP Features with Structured Data

a. Combine the extracted NLP features with structured patient demographic information, such as age, gender, and comorbidities.

b. Create a comprehensive feature set that incorporates both textual and structured data.

4. Predictive Modeling

a.Split the dataset into training and testing sets.

b. Train machine learning models, such as logistic regression, random forests, or gradient boosting, using the combined feature set to predict hospital readmissions.

c. Evaluate the performance of the models using appropriate metrics, such as accuracy, precision, recall, and F1-score.

5. Model Interpretation and Insights

a. Interpret the trained models to identify the most influential features contributing to hospital readmissions.

b. Analyze the impact of specific medical entities, sentiment, and topics on readmission risk.

c.Derive actionable insights and recommendations for reducing hospital readmissions based on the model findings.

PART III
R PROGRAMMING FOR HEALTHCARE

8 INTRODUCTION TO R PROGRAMMING

R is a powerful and versatile programming language widely used for statistical computing, data analysis, and visualization. Its extensive ecosystem of packages and libraries makes it particularly well-suited for healthcare data analysis and research. In this section, we will introduce the basics of R programming, focusing on its syntax and fundamental data structures.

8.1 Basic Syntax

R follows a simple and intuitive syntax that allows users to perform various operations and manipulate data effectively. Here are some key aspects of R's basic syntax:

8.1.1 Assignment Operator

The assignment operator in R is <-, which assigns a value to a variable.

Example: x <- 10 assigns the value 10 to the variable x.

Alternatively, the = operator can also be used for assignment, but <- is more commonly used and recommended for clarity.

8.1.2 Comments

Comments in R are used to provide explanations or

annotations within the code.

Single-line comments start with #, and everything after # on the same line is considered a comment.

Example: # This is a single-line comment

Multi-line comments are enclosed between /* and */.

Example:

/* This is a

 multi-line comment */

8.1.3 Function Calls

Functions in R are called using the syntax function_name(arguments).

Arguments are passed within the parentheses, separated by commas.

Example: sqrt(25) calls the square root function with the argument 25.

8.1.4 Packages

R has a vast collection of packages that extend its functionality for specific tasks.

Packages are installed using the install.packages() function.

Installed packages are loaded into the current R session using the library() function.

Example: library(dplyr) loads the dplyr package for data manipulation.

8.2 Data Structures

R provides several fundamental data structures to store and manipulate data. Understanding these data structures is crucial for effective data analysis and manipulation. Here are the primary data structures in R:

8.2.1 Vectors

Vectors are the most basic data structure in R, representing a sequence of elements of the same data type.

Elements in a vector are accessed using square brackets [] and a numeric index.

Example: c(1, 2, 3, 4, 5) creates a numeric vector with five elements.

8.2.2 Lists

Lists are ordered collections of objects that can contain elements of different data types.Elements in a list are accessed using double square brackets [[]] or the $ operator.

Example: list(name = "John", age = 30, is_patient = TRUE) creates a list with three named elements.

8.2.3 Matrices

Matrices are two-dimensional arrays where all elements have the same data type. Elements in a matrix are accessed using square brackets [] with row and column indices.

Example: matrix(1:9, nrow = 3, ncol = 3) creates a 3x3 matrix with elements from 1 to 9.

8.2.4 Data Frames

Data frames are two-dimensional structures similar to matrices but can contain elements of different data types in each column. Data frames are the most commonly used data structure for tabular data in R.

Elements in a data frame are accessed using square brackets [] with row and column indices or the $ operator for named columns.

Example: data.frame(name = c("John", "Alice"), age = c(30, 25), is_patient = c(TRUE, FALSE)) creates a data frame with three columns and two rows.

8.2.5 Factors

Factors are used to represent categorical variables in R. Factors are created using the factor() function, which takes a vector of values and optional levels.

Example: factor(c("male", "female", "male")) creates a factor with two levels: "male" and "female".

8.2.6 Arrays

Arrays are multi-dimensional structures that extend the

concept of matrices to higher dimensions. Elements in an array are accessed using square brackets [] with multiple indices, one for each dimension.

Example: array(1:24, dim = c(2, 3, 4)) creates a 3-dimensional array with dimensions 2x3x4.

These data structures form the foundation of data manipulation and analysis in R. They can be combined, subset, and transformed using various functions and operators to extract insights from healthcare data.

Example:

Let's consider a simple example that demonstrates the usage of basic syntax and data structures in R for healthcare data analysis.

```
# Create a data frame with patient information
patient_data <- data.frame(
  name = c("John", "Alice", "Bob", "Emma", "David"),
  age = c(45, 32, 56, 28, 61),
  gender = factor(c("Male", "Female", "Male", "Female", "Male")),
    blood_pressure = c(120, 110, 135, 95, 148),
    is_diabetic = c(FALSE, FALSE, TRUE, FALSE, TRUE)
)

# Print the patient data
print(patient_data)

# Access specific elements in the data frame
patient_data$name[3]  # Access the name of the third patient
patient_data[2, "age"]  # Access the age of the second patient

# Perform calculations on the data
mean_age <- mean(patient_data$age)
print(paste("Mean age of patients:", mean_age))

# Subset the data based on a condition
diabetic_patients <- patient_data[patient_data$is_diabetic, ]
print("Diabetic patients:")
print(diabetic_patients)

Output:
name age gender blood_pressure is_diabetic
1  John 45  Male        120      FALSE
```

```
2  Alice  32 Female       110     FALSE
3   Bob  56  Male         135     TRUE
4   Emma  28 Female        95     FALSE
5  David  61  Male         148     TRUE
[1] "Bob"
[1] 32
[1] "Mean age of patients: 44.4"
[1] "Diabetic patients:"

name age gender blood_pressure is_diabetic
3   Bob  56  Male         135     TRUE
5  David  61  Male         148     TRUE
```

In this example, we create a data frame called patient_data with information about five patients, including their name, age, gender, blood pressure, and whether they have diabetes. We demonstrate accessing specific elements in the data frame using square brackets and named columns. We also perform calculations, such as calculating the mean age of patients, and subset the data to identify diabetic patients

8.3 Control Structures and Functions

Control structures and functions are essential components of any programming language, and R is no exception. They allow you to control the flow of your code, make decisions based on conditions, and encapsulate reusable code blocks. In this section, we will explore the control structures and functions in R that are commonly used in healthcare data analysis.

8.3.1 If-Else Statements

If-else statements are used to make decisions based on conditions.

The basic syntax is:

```
if (condition) {
  # Code to execute if the condition is true
} else {
  # Code to execute if the condition is false
}
Example:
age <- 25
```

```
if (age >= 18) {
  print("Adult")
} else {
  print("Minor")
}
```

8.3.2 Loops

Loops are used to iterate over a sequence of elements or repeat a block of code multiple times. R provides two main types of loops: for loop and while loop.

for loop syntax:

```
for (variable in sequence) {
  # Code to execute for each element in the sequence
}
while loop syntax:
while (condition) {
  # Code to execute as long as the condition is true
}
Example:
# for loop
for (i in 1:5) {
  print(i)
}

# while loop
count <- 0
while (count < 3) {
  print(count)
  count <- count + 1
}
```

8.3.3 Functions

Functions are reusable code blocks that perform specific tasks. They allow you to encapsulate a series of operations and can accept arguments as input. Functions in R are defined using the function keyword followed by the function name, arguments, and the code block.

Syntax:

```
function_name <- function(arg1, arg2, ...) {
  # Code to execute
  # Optional return statement
}
Example:
calculate_bmi <- function(weight, height) {
  bmi <- weight / (height^2)
  return(bmi)
}

# Call the function
bmi_result <- calculate_bmi(weight = 75, height = 1.8)
print(bmi_result)
```

8.3.4 Apply Family of Functions

R provides a family of apply functions that allow you to apply a function to elements of a data structure. The most commonly used apply functions are apply(), lapply(), sapply(), and mapply().

apply() is used to apply a function over the margins of an array or matrix.

lapply() applies a function to each element of a list or vector and returns a list.

sapply() is similar to lapply() but simplifies the output to a vector or matrix if possible.

mapply() applies a function to the corresponding elements of multiple lists or vectors.

Example:

```
# Using lapply() to calculate BMI for a list of patients
patient_data <- list(
  list(weight = 75, height = 1.8),
  list(weight = 68, height = 1.6),
  list(weight = 82, height = 1.75)
)

bmi_results <- lapply(patient_data, function(patient) {
  bmi <- patient$weight / (patient$height^2)
  return(bmi)
```

```
})
```

```
print(bmi_results)
```

These control structures and functions provide the necessary tools to control the flow of your code, make decisions based on conditions, iterate over data, and create reusable code blocks. They are fundamental to any data analysis task in R, including healthcare data analysis.

Example:

Let's consider an example that demonstrates the usage of control structures and functions in R for analyzing patient data.

```
# Function to categorize blood pressure
categorize_bp <- function(bp) {
  if (bp < 120) {
    return("Normal")
  } else if (bp >= 120 && bp < 140) {
    return("Prehypertension")
  } else if (bp >= 140 && bp < 160) {
    return("Stage 1 Hypertension")
  } else {
    return("Stage 2 Hypertension")
  }
}

# Patient data
patient_data <- data.frame(
  name = c("John", "Alice", "Bob", "Emma", "David"),
  age = c(45, 32, 56, 28, 61),
  blood_pressure = c(120, 110, 135, 95, 148)
)

# Categorize blood pressure for each patient
bp_categories <- sapply(patient_data$blood_pressure, categorize_bp)

# Add the blood pressure category to the patient data
patient_data$bp_category <- bp_categories

# Print the updated patient data
print(patient_data)
```

```
# Count the number of patients in each blood pressure category
bp_counts <- table(patient_data$bp_category)
print(bp_counts)
```

```
Output:
  name      age blood_pressure  bp_category
1 John       45      120            Prehypertension
2 Alice 32     110    Normal
3 Bob        56     135            Prehypertension
4 Emma 28      95               Normal
5 David 61       148    Stage1 Hypertension


Normal   Prehypertension Stage 1 Hypertension
   2         2                 1
```

In this example, we define a function called categorize_bp() that takes a blood pressure value as input and returns the corresponding blood pressure category based on the specified ranges. We use if-else statements within the function to determine the appropriate category.

We have a data frame called patient_data that contains information about five patients, including their name, age, and blood pressure. We use the sapply() function to apply the categorize_bp() function to each blood pressure value in the patient_data$blood_pressure vector. The resulting blood

pressure categories are stored in the bp_categories vector. We then add the blood pressure categories to the patient_data data frame as a new column called bp_category. Finally, we print the updated patient data and use the table() function to count the number of patients in each blood pressure category.

This example showcases how control structures (if-else statements) and functions (categorize_bp()) can be used together to analyze and categorize healthcare data in R. The apply family of functions, such as sapply(), allows us to efficiently apply the categorization function to each element of the blood pressure vector

8.4 Packages and Libraries in R

R has a vast ecosystem of packages and libraries that extend its functionality and provide specialized tools for various domains, including healthcare data analysis. Packages are collections of functions, data, and documentation that can be installed and loaded into an R session. In this section, we will explore some essential packages and libraries commonly used in healthcare data analysis.

8.4.1 Base R Packages

R comes with a set of built-in packages that provide core functionality for data manipulation, statistical analysis, and visualization.

Some notable base R packages include:

stats: Provides functions for statistical calculations and modeling.

graphics: Offers functions for creating various types of plots and charts.

utils: Contains utility functions for data input/output, package management, and more.

These packages are automatically loaded when you start an R session.

8.4.2 Installing and Loading Package

To use additional packages, you need to install them first and then load them into your R session. To install a package, use the install.packages() function, providing the package name in quotes.

Example: install.packages("dplyr") installs the dplyr package.

Once installed, you can load a package using the library() function.

Example: library(dplyr) loads the dplyr package into the current R session.

8.4.3 Essential Packages for Healthcare Data Analysis

dplyr: Provides a set of functions for efficient data manipulation and transformation.

tidyr: Offers functions for data tidying and reshaping, making data easier to work with.

ggplot2: A powerful package for creating attractive and customizable visualizations.

readr: Provides functions for reading and parsing tabular data from various file formats.

lubridate: Helps in working with dates and times, making date-based operations easier.

stringr: Offers functions for string manipulation and text processing.

caret: A comprehensive package for machine learning and predictive modeling.

survival: Provides functions for survival analysis and modeling time-to-event data.

pROC: Offers tools for receiver operating characteristic (ROC) curve analysis.

ggpubr: Enhances the functionality of ggplot2 with additional themes and utilities.

8.4.4 Domain-Specific Packages

R has numerous packages tailored for specific domains within healthcare, such as genomics, epidemiology, and clinical trials.

Examples of domain-specific packages include:

Bioconductor: A collection of packages for bioinformatics and genomic data analysis.

epiR: Provides functions for epidemiological data analysis and modeling.

survival: Offers functions for survival analysis and time-to-event data.

meta: Provides tools for meta-analysis and evidence synthesis.

ClinicalTrialSummary: Generates summary tables and visualizations for clinical trial data.

These packages offer specialized functions and datasets specific to their respective domains.

8.4.5 Package Documentation and Help

Each package comes with documentation and help files that provide information on its functions, usage, and examples. To access the documentation for a specific function, use the help() or ? function followed by the function name.

Example: help(filter) or ?filter opens the documentation for the filter() function from the dplyr package.

The documentation includes a description of the function, its arguments, and examples of how to use it. You can also access the package vignettes and manuals using the browseVignettes() function.

Example:

Let's consider an example that demonstrates the usage of packages in R for healthcare data analysis.

```r
# Install and load required packages
install.packages("dplyr")
install.packages("ggplot2")
library(dplyr)
library(ggplot2)

# Load example dataset
data(mtcars)

# Data manipulation using dplyr
filtered_data <- mtcars %>%
  filter(mpg > 20) %>%
  select(mpg, cyl, hp)

# Print the filtered data
print(filtered_data)

# Data visualization using ggplot2
ggplot(filtered_data, aes(x = cyl, y = mpg)) +
  geom_point() +
  labs(x = "Number of Cylinders", y = "Miles per Gallon",
    title = "Fuel Efficiency by Number of Cylinders")
```

Output:

	mpg	cyl	hp
Mazda RX4	21.0	6	110
Mazda RX4 Wag	21.0	6	110
Datsun 710	22.8	4	93
Hornet 4 Drive	21.4	6	110

Valiant	18.1	6	105
Merc 240D	24.4	4	62
Merc 230	22.8	4	95
Fiat 128	32.4	4	66
Honda Civic	30.4	4	52
Toyota Corolla	33.9	4	65
Toyota Corona	21.5	4	97
Fiat X1-9	27.3	4	66
Porsche 914-2	26.0	4	91
Lotus Europa	30.4	4	113
Volvo 142E	21.4	4	109

In this example, we install and load the dplyr and ggplot2 packages, which are essential for data manipulation and visualization, respectively.

We load the mtcars dataset, which is a built-in dataset in R, for demonstration purposes. Using the dplyr package, we perform data manipulation operations such as filtering the data to include only cars with mpg greater than 20 and selecting specific columns (mpg, cyl, hp) using the filter() and select() functions.

Next, we use the ggplot2 package to create a scatter plot visualizing the relationship between the number of cylinders and fuel efficiency (mpg). We specify the data, aesthetics (x and y variables), and add a point geometry using geom_point(). We also customize the plot labels using the labs() function.

The resulting plot provides a visual representation of the filtered data, showing the relationship between the number of cylinders and fuel efficiency.

This example demonstrates how packages like dplyr and ggplot2 can be used together to perform data manipulation and visualization tasks in R. Similar principles can be applied to healthcare data analysis, where you can leverage domain-specific packages to preprocess, analyze, and visualize healthcare data effectively

.

9 STATISTICAL ANALYSIS AND VISUALIZATION WITH R

Statistical analysis and visualization are crucial components of healthcare data analysis. R provides a rich set of functions and packages for performing various statistical tests, calculating descriptive statistics, and creating informative visualizations. In this section, we will explore how to conduct descriptive statistics and hypothesis testing using R.

9.1 Descriptive Statistics

Descriptive statistics help summarize and describe the main features of a dataset. They provide insights into the central tendency, variability, and distribution of the data. R offers several functions for calculating descriptive statistics:

mean(): Calculates the arithmetic mean of a numeric vector.

Example: mean(patient_ages)

median(): Calculates the median value of a numeric vector.

Example: median(patient_weights)

sd(): Calculates the standard deviation of a numeric vector.

Example: sd(patient_heights)

var(): Calculates the variance of a numeric vector.

Example: var(patient_blood_pressure)

min() and max(): Find the minimum and maximum values in a numeric vector.

Example: min(patient_ages), max(patient_ages)

quantile(): Calculates the specified quantiles of a numeric vector.

Example: quantile(patient_ages, probs = c(0.25, 0.5, 0.75))

summary(): Provides a summary of a dataset, including minimum, maximum, quartiles, and mean.

Example: summary(patient_data)

These functions allow you to quickly obtain key descriptive statistics for your healthcare data, giving you an overview of the data's characteristics.

Example:

```
# Patient data
patient_data <- data.frame(
  age = c(45, 32, 56, 28, 61, 50, 39, 42, 37, 52),
  weight = c(75, 68, 82, 60, 90, 85, 72, 78, 69, 88),
  height = c(1.75, 1.62, 1.80, 1.55, 1.85, 1.78, 1.65, 1.73, 1.60, 1.82)
)

# Calculate descriptive statistics
mean_age <- mean(patient_data$age)
```

```
median_weight <- median(patient_data$weight)
sd_height <- sd(patient_data$height)
min_age <- min(patient_data$age)
max_weight <- max(patient_data$weight)

# Print the results
cat("Mean age:", mean_age, "\n")
cat("Median weight:", median_weight, "\n")
cat("Standard deviation of height:", sd_height, "\n")
cat("Minimum age:", min_age, "\n")
cat("Maximum weight:", max_weight, "\n")

# Summary of the patient data
summary(patient_data)
```

Output:
Mean age: 44.2
Median weight: 76.5
Standard deviation of height: 0.1032796
Minimum age: 28
Maximum weight: 90

```
 age              weight        height
Min:28.00           Min.:60.00  Min.  :1.550
1st Qu:37.75   1st Qu:69.75  1st Qu.:1.625
Median :43.50  Median:76.50  Median :1.740
Mean   :44.20  Mean:76.70  Mean   :1.715
3rd Qu.:51.25  3rd Qu:84.25 3rd Qu.:1.808
Max.:61.00      Max.: 90.00 Max.   :1.850
```

9.2 Hypothesis Testing

Hypothesis testing is a statistical method used to make decisions based on sample data. It involves formulating a null hypothesis (H0) and an alternative hypothesis (H1), and then using statistical tests to determine whether to reject or fail to reject the null hypothesis. R provides functions for various statistical tests commonly used in healthcare research.

9.2.1 t-test

Used to compare the means of two groups or to test if a sample mean differs from a known population mean.
t.test() function is used for performing t-tests.
Example: t.test(group1_data, group2_data, var.equal = TRUE)

9.2.2 ANOVA (Analysis of Variance)

Used to compare the means of three or more groups.
aov() function is used for performing one-way ANOVA.
Example: aov(response ~ group, data = dataset)

9.2.3 Chi-square test

Used to test the association between categorical variables.
chisq.test() function is used for performing chi-square tests.
Example: chisq.test(contingency_table)

9.2.4 Wilcoxon rank-sum test

A non-parametric alternative to the two-sample t-test,
used when the assumptions of normality are not met.
wilcox.test() function is used for performing Wilcoxon rank-sum tests.
Example: wilcox.test(group1_data, group2_data)

9.2.5 Kruskal-Wallis test

A non-parametric alternative to one-way ANOVA,
used when the assumptions of normality are not met.
kruskal.test() function is used for performing Kruskal-Wallis tests.
Example: kruskal.test(response ~ group, data = dataset)
These are just a few examples of the statistical tests available in R. It's important to choose the appropriate test based on the research question, study design, and the nature of the data.

Example:
```r
# Patient groups
group1_bp <- c(120, 125, 118, 130, 122)
group2_bp <- c(135, 140, 138, 145, 142)

# Perform a two-sample t-test
t_test_result <- t.test(group1_bp, group2_bp, var.equal = TRUE)
print(t_test_result)

# Patient data for ANOVA
patient_data <- data.frame(
    group = c(rep("A", 5), rep("B", 5), rep("C",5)),
    response = c(2.5, 3.2, 2.8, 3.0, 2.7, 3.5, 3.8, 3.6, 3.9, 3.7, 4.2, 4.5,
```

```
4.3, 4.1, 4.0)
)

# Perform one-way ANOVA
anova_result <- aov(response ~ group, data = patient_data)
print(summary(anova_result))
```

Output:
```
   Welch Two Sample t-test
data:  group1_bp and group2_bp
t = -8.6603, df = 8, p-value = 2.681e-05
alternative hypothesis: true difference in means is not equal to 0
95 percent confidence interval:
 -21.35975 -12.64025
sample estimates:
mean of x mean of y
   123.0    140.0


        Df Sum Sq Mean Sq F value   Pr(>F)
group     2  5.113   2.557   106.5 2.52e-08 ***
Residuals 12  0.288   0.024           ---
Signif. codes:  0 '***' 0.001 '**' 0.01 '*' 0.05
'.' 0.1 ' ' 1
```

In the first example, we perform a two-sample t-test to compare the mean blood pressure between two groups (group1_bp and group2_bp). The t.test() function is used, and the results show a significant difference in means between the two groups (p-value < 0.05).

In the second example, we have patient data with three groups (A, B, C) and their corresponding response values. We perform a one-way ANOVA using the aov() function to test if there are significant differences in the mean response values among the three groups. The ANOVA results indicate a highly significant difference among the groups (p-value < 0.001)

9.3 ggplot2 for Data Visualization

Data visualization is an essential part of healthcare data analysis, as it helps to communicate complex information in a clear and intuitive way. R provides a powerful package called ggplot2 for creating high-quality and customizable visualizations. In this section, we will explore how to use ggplot2 to create various types of plots commonly used in healthcare research.

9.3.1 Scatter plot

Used to visualize the relationship between two continuous variables.

geom_point() function is used to create scatter plots.

Example:
```
ggplot(data, aes(x = age, y = weight)) +
  geom_point()
```

9.3.2 Line plot

Used to display trends or changes over time.

geom_line() function is used to create line plots.

Example:
```
ggplot(data, aes(x = year, y = cases)) +
  geom_line()
```

9.3.3 Bar plot

Used to compare values across different categories.

geom_bar() function is used to create bar plots.

Example:
```
ggplot(data, aes(x = group, y = count)) +
  geom_bar(stat = "identity")
```

9.3.5 Histogram

Used to visualize the distribution of a single continuous variable.

geom_histogram() function is used to create histograms.

Example:
```
ggplot(data, aes(x = age)) +
  geom_histogram(binwidth = 5)
```

9.3.6 Box plot

Used to display the distribution and summary statistics of a continuous variable across different categories.

geom_boxplot() function is used to create box plots.

Example:
```
ggplot(data, aes(x = group, y = value)) +
  geom_boxplot()
```

9.3.7 Faceting

Used to create multiple plots based on different subsets of the data.

facet_wrap() or facet_grid() functions are used for faceting.

Example:
```
ggplot(data, aes(x = age, y = weight)) +
  geom_point() +
  facet_wrap(~ gender)
```

9.3.8 Customization

ggplot2 provides a wide range of options for customizing plots, including colors, labels, scales, and themes.

Example:
```
ggplot(data, aes(x = age, y = weight, color = gender)) +
geom_point() +
  labs(title = "Weight vs. Age", x = "Age (years)", y =
"Weight (kg)") +
scale_color_manual(values = c("blue", "red")) + theme_minimal()
```

These are just a few examples of the visualizations that can be created using ggplot2. The package offers a flexible and layered approach to building plots, allowing you to combine different geometries, aesthetics, and transformations to create complex and informative visualizations.

Example:
```
# Install and load the ggplot2 package
install.packages("ggplot2")
library(ggplot2)
```

```r
# Create example data
data <- data.frame(
  group = c(rep("A", 50), rep("B", 50)),
  age = c(rnorm(50, mean = 40, sd = 5), rnorm(50, mean = 45, sd =
6)),
weight = c(rnorm(50, mean = 70, sd = 10), rnorm(50, mean = 75, sd
= 12)),
gender = c(rep(c("Male", "Female"), each = 25), rep(c("Male",
"Female"), each = 25))
)


# Scatter plot with faceting by gender
ggplot(data, aes(x = age, y = weight, color = group)) +
  geom_point() +
  facet_wrap(~ gender) +
  labs(title = "Weight vs. Age by Gender", x = "Age     (years)", y =
"Weight (kg)") +
    scale_color_manual(values = c("blue", "red")) +
  theme_minimal()

# Box plot of weight by group
ggplot(data, aes(x = group, y = weight)) +
  geom_boxplot() +
      labs(title = "Weight Distribution by Group", x = "Group", y
    = "Weight (kg)") +
  theme_minimal()
```

In this example, we first install and load the ggplot2 package. Then, we create an example dataset called data with columns for group, age, weight, and gender.

Using ggplot2, we create two visualizations:
A scatter plot of weight vs. age, faceted by gender. We use geom_point() to create the scatter plot, facet_wrap() to create separate plots for each gender, and customize the plot with labels, colors, and a minimalistic theme.
A box plot of weight distribution by group. We use geom_boxplot() to create the box plot, and customize the plot with labels and a minimalistic theme.
These examples demonstrate how ggplot2 can be used to create informative and visually appealing plots for healthcare data analysis

Case Study 1: Analyzing Clinical Trial Data

Objective:

In this case study, we will analyze data from a clinical trial that investigated the efficacy of a new drug for treating hypertension. The goal is to compare the blood pressure reduction between the treatment and placebo groups and determine if there is a significant difference.

Dataset:

The dataset contains information on 200 patients, including their unique ID, age, gender, baseline blood pressure, post-treatment blood pressure, and treatment group (0 for placebo, 1 for treatment).

Steps:

a. Load the dataset into R and perform data cleaning and preprocessing if necessary.

b. Explore the dataset using descriptive statistics and visualizations.

c. Compare the baseline characteristics between the treatment and placebo groups.

d. Calculate the mean blood pressure reduction for each group.

e. Perform a two-sample t-test to determine if there is a significant difference in blood pressure reduction between the two groups.

f. Visualize the results using appropriate plots, such as box plots or scatter plots.

g. Interpret the findings and draw conclusions based on the statistical analysis.

Example code snippets:

```
# Load the dataset
data <- read.csv("clinical_trial_data.csv")

# Descriptive statistics
summary(data)
```

```
# Compare baseline characteristics
table(data$treatment, data$gender)
boxplot(age ~ treatment, data = data)

# Calculate mean blood pressure reduction
bp_reduction <- data$baseline_bp - data$post_treatment_bp
tapply(bp_reduction, data$treatment, mean)

# Perform two-sample t-test
t.test(bp_reduction ~ treatment, data = data)

# Visualize results
boxplot(bp_reduction ~ treatment, data = data,
xlab = "Treatment Group", ylab = "Blood Pressure Reduction")
```

Case Study 2: Predicting Hospital Readmission

Objective

In this case study, we aim to build a predictive model to identify patients who are at high risk of hospital readmission within 30 days of discharge. Healthcare providers can allocate resources and interventions to reduce readmission rates and improve patient outcomes by accurately predicting readmission risk.

Dataset

The dataset contains information on 5,000 patients, including demographic variables (age, gender), clinical variables (comorbidities, length of stay), and readmission status (1 for readmitted within 30 days, 0 for not readmitted).

Steps

    a. Load the dataset into R and perform data exploration and preprocessing.

    b. Split the dataset into training and testing sets.

    c. Build a logistic regression model using the training set to predict readmission risk.

    d. Evaluate the model's performance using

appropriate metrics such as accuracy, precision, recall, and F1 score.

e.Identify the most important predictors of readmission risk.

f. Validate the model using the testing set and assess its generalizability.

g. Interpret the model coefficients and discuss the implications for clinical practice.

Example code snippets:

```
# Load the dataset
data <- read.csv("hospital_readmission_data.csv")

# Split the dataset into training and testing sets
set.seed(123)
train_indices <- sample(1:nrow(data), 0.7 * nrow(data))
train_data <- data[train_indices, ]
test_data <- data[-train_indices, ]

# Build logistic regression model
model <- glm(readmission ~ ., data = train_data, family = "binomial")
summary(model)

# Evaluate model performance
predicted_prob <- predict(model, test_data, type = "response")
predicted_class <- ifelse(predicted_prob > 0.5, 1, 0)
confusionMatrix(table(predicted_class, test_data$readmission))

# Identify important predictors
ggplot(data = coef_df, aes(x = reorder(term, estimate), y = estimate)) +
  geom_point() +
  coord_flip() +
  labs(x = "Variable", y = "Coefficient Estimate")
```

Case Study 3: Analyzing Patient Survival Data

Objective

In this case study, we will analyze survival data of patients diagnosed with a specific type of cancer. The goal is to investigate the factors that influence patient survival and to visualize survival curves for different subgroups.

Dataset

The dataset contains information on 500 cancer patients, including their unique ID, age at diagnosis, gender, tumor stage (I, II, III, IV), treatment received (surgery, chemotherapy, radiation), and survival time (in months). The dataset also includes a censoring indicator variable, where 1 indicates that the patient's survival time is censored (i.e., the patient was still alive at the end of the study or lost to follow-up), and 0 indicates that the patient's survival time is complete (i.e., the patient died during the study period).

Steps

a. Load the dataset into R and perform data cleaning and preprocessing if necessary.

b. Explore the dataset using descriptive statistics and visualizations.

c. Create a survival object using the Surv() function from the survival package.

d. Fit a Cox proportional hazards model to identify significant predictors of patient survival.

e. Plot the Kaplan-Meier survival curves for different subgroups (e.g., by tumor stage or treatment received).

f. Interpret the results of the Cox model and the survival curves.

g. Discuss the implications of the findings for clinical practice and patient care.

Example code snippets:

```r
# Load the dataset
data <- read.csv("cancer_survival_data.csv")

# Create survival object
library(survival)
surv_object<-Surv(data$survival_time, data$censoring_indicator)

# Fit Cox proportional hazards model
cox_model <- coxph(surv_object ~ age + gender + tumor_stage + treatment, data = data)
summary(cox_model)
```

```
# Plot Kaplan-Meier survival curves by tumor stage
fit <- survfit(surv_object ~ tumor_stage, data = data)
ggsurvplot(fit, data = data,
       risk.table = TRUE,
       pval = TRUE,
       conf.int = TRUE,
       legend.labs = c("Stage I", "Stage II", "Stage III", "Stage IV"),
              xlab = "Time (months)", ylab = "Survival
Probability")
```

These case studies demonstrate the application of R in different healthcare data analysis scenarios, including clinical trial analysis, predictive modeling for hospital readmission, and survival analysis for cancer patients. Each case study involves specific objectives, datasets, and statistical techniques commonly used in healthcare research.

10 BIOINFORMATICS AND GENOMIC DATA ANALYSIS WITH R

Bioinformatics is an interdisciplinary field that combines computer science, statistics, and biology to analyze and interpret biological data, particularly genomic data. R provides a rich ecosystem of packages and tools for bioinformatics and genomic data analysis. In this section, we will explore the basics of bioinformatics and how R can be used to handle and analyze genomic data.

10.1 Introduction to Bioinformatics

Bioinformatics involves the application of computational methods to manage, analyze, and interpret biological data. It plays a crucial role in modern biology and has been instrumental in advancing our understanding of genomics, proteomics, and systems biology. Some key areas of bioinformatics include:

a. Sequence analysis: Analyzing DNA, RNA, and protein sequences to identify patterns, motifs, and functional elements.

b. Genome assembly and annotation: Reconstructing complete genomes from sequencing reads and identifying genes, regulatory regions, and other genomic features.

3. Gene expression analysis: Quantifying and comparing

gene expression levels across different conditions or samples using microarray or RNA-seq data.

4. Protein structure and function prediction: Predicting the three-dimensional structure and function of proteins based on their amino acid sequences.

5. Pathway and network analysis: Studying the interactions and relationships between genes, proteins, and other biological entities to understand cellular processes and disease mechanisms.

R provides a wide range of packages and tools specifically designed for bioinformatics tasks. Some popular bioinformatics packages in R include:

Biostrings: Provides tools for working with biological strings, such as DNA, RNA, and amino acid sequences.

BSgenome: Offers infrastructure for efficient representation and manipulation of full genomes and their annotations.

Rsamtools: Provides an interface for reading and manipulating sequence alignment data in SAM/BAM format.

GenomicRanges: Defines general purpose containers for storing genomic ranges and associated annotations.

DESeq2 and edgeR: Widely used packages for differential gene expression analysis of RNA-seq data.

limma: Provides tools for analyzing gene expression data from microarrays and RNA-seq experiments.

Example:

```
# Install and load the Biostrings package
install.packages("Biostrings")
library(Biostrings)

# Create a DNA sequence
dna_seq<- DNAString("ATGCATGCATGCATGC")

# Compute the reverse complement of the DNA sequence
rev_comp <- reverseComplement(dna_seq)
print(rev_comp)

# Translate the DNA sequence into a protein sequence
```

```
protein_seq <- translate(dna_seq)
print(protein_seq)

# Perform pairwise alignment of two DNA sequences
seq1 <- DNAString("ATGCATGC")
seq2 <- DNAString("ATGCCTGC")
alignment <- pairwiseAlignment(seq1, seq2)
print(alignment)

16-letter DNAString instance
seq: GCATGCATGCATGCAT

5-letter AAString instance
seq: MHACI

Global PairwiseAlignmentsSingleSubject (1 of 1)
pattern: [1] ATGCATGC
subject: [1] ATGCCTGC
score: 13

Global PairwiseAlignmentsSingleSubject (1 of 1)
pattern: [1] ATGCATGC
subject: [1] ATGCCTGC
score: 13
```

In this example, we use the Biostrings package to work with DNA sequences. We create a DNA sequence, compute its reverse complement, translate it into a protein sequence, and perform pairwise alignment between two DNA sequences.

These are just a few examples of the capabilities of R in bioinformatics. R provides a comprehensive set of tools and packages for handling and analyzing various types of biological data, making it a powerful platform for bioinformatics research

10.2 Bioconductor for Genomic Data Analysis

Bioconductor is an open-source software project for the analysis and comprehension of genomic data. It is built on top of the R programming language and provides a wide range of tools and packages specifically designed for bioinformatics and genomic data analysis.

Bioconductor offers a consistent and integrated framework for working with genomic data, making it a go-to resource for bioinformaticians and researchers in the field.

Key features of Bioconductor include:

1. Extensive collection of packages: Bioconductor hosts over 2,000 packages covering various aspects of genomic data analysis, including sequence analysis, microarray analysis, RNA-seq analysis, proteomics, and more.

2. Standardized data structures: Bioconductor defines standard data structures, such as GRanges and SummarizedExperiment, which provide a consistent way to store and manipulate genomic data and metadata.

3. Documentation and tutorials: Bioconductor provides extensive documentation, vignettes, and tutorials for its packages, making it easier for users to learn and apply the tools effectively.

4. Active community and support: Bioconductor has a large and active community of developers and users who contribute to the project, provide support, and share knowledge through mailing lists, forums, and conferences.

To get started with Bioconductor, you need to install it in your R environment. You can use the following commands to install Bioconductor:

```
# Install BiocManager
install.packages("BiocManager")

# Install Bioconductor packages
BiocManager::install(c("GenomicRanges",          "Biostrings",
"DESeq2"))
Here's an example of using Bioconductor packages for genomic
data analysis:
# Load required packages
library(GenomicRanges)
library(Biostrings)
library(DESeq2)

# Create a GRanges object representing genomic ranges
gr <- GRanges(seqnames = c("chr1", "chr1", "chr2"),
```

```
  ranges = IRanges(start = c(100, 200, 300), end = c(150, 250,
  350)),
            strand = c("+", "-", "+"))

# Perform operations on genomic ranges
gr_subset <- gr[seqnames(gr) == "chr1"]
gr_width <- width(gr)

# Load a FASTA file containing DNA sequences
dna_sequences <- readDNAStringSet("sequences.fasta")

# Perform sequence analysis
gc_content <- letterFrequency(dna_sequences, "GC", as.prob =
TRUE)

# Perform differential expression analysis using DESeq2
dds <- DESeqDataSetFromMatrix(countData = count_matrix,
colData = sample_info, design = ~ condition)
dds <- DESeq(dds)
results <- results(dds, contrast = c("condition", "treated",
"control"))
```

In this example, we demonstrate the usage of several Bioconductor packages:

1. GenomicRanges: We create a GRanges object to represent genomic ranges and perform operations like subsetting and computing the width of the ranges.

2. Biostrings: We load DNA sequences from a FASTA file using the readDNAStringSet function and compute the GC content of the sequences using the letterFrequency function.

3. DESeq2: We perform differential expression analysis using the DESeq2 package. We create a DESeqDataSet object from a count matrix and sample information, run the DESeq2 analysis, and extract the results.

These are just a few examples of the capabilities of Bioconductor packages. Bioconductor provides a rich ecosystem of tools for various genomic data analysis tasks, including gene expression analysis, ChIP-seq analysis, variant calling, pathway analysis, and more

Case Study 1: Analyzing Gene Expression Data

Objective:

In this case study, we will analyze gene expression data from a microarray experiment to identify differentially expressed genes between two conditions (e.g., treated vs. control). We will use the limma package from Bioconductor to perform the analysis and visualize the results.

Dataset:

The dataset for this case study consists of gene expression data from a microarray experiment. The data is stored in a text file with rows representing genes and columns representing samples. The first column contains gene identifiers, and the remaining columns contain expression values for each sample. The dataset includes samples from two conditions: treated and control.

Steps:

1. Install and load the required Bioconductor packages:

```
# Install Bioconductor packages
BiocManager::install(c("limma", "edgeR"))

# Load the packages
library(limma)
library(edgeR)
```

2. Read the gene expression data into R:

```
# Read the gene expression data
data <- read.delim("gene_expression_data.txt", stringsAsFactors = FALSE)
```

3. Preprocess the data:

Extract the gene identifiers and expression values
Convert the expression values to a matrix
Create a sample information data frame

```
# Extract gene identifiers and expression values
gene_ids <- data[, 1]
```

```r
expression_matrix <- as.matrix(data[, -1])

# Create a sample information data frame
sample_info <- data.frame(
  Sample = colnames(expression_matrix),
  Condition = c(rep("Treated", 3), rep("Control", 3)))
```

4. Perform differential expression analysis using limma:

Create a design matrix specifying the conditions
Fit a linear model to the data
Estimate contrast and calculate moderated t-statistics
Adjust p-values for multiple testing

```r
# Create a design matrix
design_matrix <- model.matrix(~Condition, data = sample_info)

# Fit a linear model
fit <- lmFit(expression_matrix, design_matrix)

# Estimate contrast and calculate moderated t-statistics
contrast_matrix <- makeContrasts(TreatedvsControl = Treated - Control, levels = design_matrix)
fit2 <- contrasts.fit(fit, contrast_matrix)
fit2 <- eBayes(fit2)

# Extract results and adjust p-values
results <- topTable(fit2, coef = "TreatedvsControl", adjust.method = "BH", number = Inf)
```

5. Visualize the results:

Create a volcano plot to visualize differentially expressed genes
Create a heatmap to visualize the expression patterns of top differentially expressed genes

```r
# Create a volcano plot
plot(results$logFC, -log10(results$P.Value),
    xlab = "Log2 Fold Change", ylab = "-log10(P-Value)",
    main = "Volcano Plot")
abline(h = -log10(0.05), col = "red", lty = 2)

# Create a heatmap of top differentially expressed genes
top_genes <- rownames(results)[1:50]
heatmap_data <- expression_matrix[top_genes, ]
```

```
heatmap(heatmap_data, scale = "row",
col = colorRampPalette(c("blue", "white", "red"))(100),
main = "Heatmap of Top Differentially Expressed Genes")
```

6. Interpret the results:
Examine the differentially expressed genes (significant p-values and fold changes)
Consider the biological significance and relevance of the identified genes
Investigate the functions and pathways associated with the differentially expressed genes

Results:

The analysis will provide a list of differentially expressed genes between the treated and control conditions. The volcano plot will visualize the significance and magnitude of gene expression changes, with significant genes highlighted. The heatmap will display the expression patterns of the top differentially expressed genes across the samples.

Case Study 2: Analyzing RNA-Seq Data for Differential Gene Expression

Objective:

In this case study, we will analyze RNA-seq data to identify differentially expressed genes between two conditions (e.g., disease vs. control). We will use the DESeq2 package from Bioconductor to perform the analysis and visualize the results.

Dataset:

The dataset for this case study consists of RNA-seq count data, where each row represents a gene and each column represents a sample. The count matrix is stored in a CSV file named "rnaseq_counts.csv". Additionally, we have a metadata file named "sample_metadata.csv" that contains information about each sample, including the condition (disease or control).

Steps:
1. Install and load the required Bioconductor packages:

```
# Install Bioconductor packages
BiocManager::install(c("DESeq2", "ggplot2"))

# Load the packages
library(DESeq2)
library(ggplot2)
```

2. Read the RNA-seq count data and sample metadata into R:

```
# Read the count matrix
count_matrix <- read.csv("rnaseq_counts.csv", row.names = 1)
# Read the sample metadata
sample_metadata    <-    read.csv("sample_metadata.csv",
row.names = 1)
```

3. Create a DESeqDataSet object:

```
# Create a DESeqDataSet object
dds <- DESeqDataSetFromMatrix(countData= count_matrix,
colData = sample_metadata,
design = ~ Condition)
```

4. Perform differential expression analysis using DESeq2:

```
# Run DESeq2 analysis
dds <- DESeq(dds)

# Extract the results
res <- results(dds, contrast = c("Condition", "Disease",
"Control"))
```

5. Visualize the results:
Create an MA plot to visualize the differentially expressed genes
Create a heatmap of the top differentially expressed genes

```
# Create an MA plot
plotMA(res, ylim = c(-5, 5))
```

```
# Create a heatmap of the top differentially expressed genes
top_genes <- rownames(res)[order(res$padj)[1:50]]
normalized_counts <- counts(dds, normalized = TRUE)
heatmap_data <- normalized_counts[top_genes, ]
pheatmap(heatmap_data, scale = "row", show_rownames =
FALSE)
```

6. Interpret the results:

Examine the differentially expressed genes (significant adjusted p-values and log2 fold changes)

Investigate the biological functions and pathways associated with the identified genes

Results:

The analysis will provide a list of differentially expressed genes between the disease and control conditions. The MA plot will visualize the relationship between the log2 fold changes and the average expression levels, highlighting significantly differentially expressed genes. The heatmap will display the expression patterns of the top differentially expressed genes across the samples.

Case Study 3: Genome-Wide Association Study (GWAS) Analysis

Objective:

In this case study, we will perform a genome-wide association study (GWAS) to identify genetic variants associated with a particular trait or disease. We will use the SNPRelate package from Bioconductor to perform quality control, principal component analysis (PCA), and association testing.

Dataset:

The dataset for this case study consists of genotype data in the form of a PLINK binary file format (.bed, .bim, .fam files). The genotype data includes information about single nucleotide polymorphisms (SNPs) for a set of individuals. Additionally, we have a phenotype file named "phenotype.txt" that contains the trait or disease status for each individual.

Steps:
1.Install and load the required Bioconductor packages:

```
# Install Bioconductor packages
BiocManager::install(c("SNPRelate", "ggplot2"))

# Load the packages
library(SNPRelate)
library(ggplot2)
```

2. Read the genotype data and phenotype data into R:

```
# Read the genotype data
snp_data <- snpgdsBED2GDS("genotype")

# Read the phenotype data
phenotype_data <- read.table("phenotype.txt", header = TRUE)
```

3. Perform quality control:

Filter out SNPs with low call rates and minor allele frequencies
Filter out individuals with low genotyping rates
Check for gender mismatches

```
# Perform quality control
snp_data <- snpgdsQC(snp_data, sample.id = phenotype_data$Sample_ID)
snp_data <- snpgdsLDpruning(snp_data, method = "corr", slide.max.bp = 10000, ld.threshold = 0.2)
```

4. Perform principal component analysis (PCA) to identify population structure:

```
# Perform PCA
pca <- snpgdsPCA(snp_data, num.thread = 2)

# Plot the PCA results
plot(pca$eigenvect[, 1], pca$eigenvect[, 2], xlab = "PC1", ylab = "PC2")
```

5. Perform association testing:

Conduct a single-SNP association test using a linear or logistic regression model

Adjust for population structure using the PCA results

```
# Perform association testing
gwas_results          <-          snpgdsSNPAssociation(snp_data,
phenotype_data$Trait,    method   =    "linear",    covar   =
pca$eigenvect[, 1:10])

# Visualize the GWAS results
manhattan_plot <- ggplot(gwas_results, aes(x = Chromosome, y
= -log10(P_value))) +
  geom_point() +
  xlab("Chromosome") +
  ylab("-log10(P-value)")
print(manhattan_plot)
```

6. Interpret the results:

Identify SNPs that reach genome-wide significance (p-value < 5e-8)

Investigate the genes closest to the significant SNPs

Explore the biological functions and pathways associated with the identified genes

Results

The analysis will provide a list of SNPs associated with the trait or disease of interest. The Manhattan plot will visualize the association results, highlighting SNPs that reach genome-wide significance. The PCA plot will display the population structure and identify potential confounding factors

PART IV: OTHER PROGRAMMING LANGUAGES AND APPLICATIONS

11 JAVA PROGRAMMING FOR HEALTHCARE SOFTWARE DEVELOPMENT

Java is a popular programming language known for its

robustness, scalability, and cross-platform compatibility. It is widely used in various domains, including healthcare software development. Java's object-oriented programming paradigm, extensive libraries, and strong community support make it a reliable choice for building healthcare applications.

11.1 Introduction to Java Programming

Java is an object-oriented programming language that follows the "write once, run anywhere" principle. It means that Java code written on one platform can be executed on any other platform that supports Java without the need for recompilation. This platform independence is achieved through the Java Virtual Machine (JVM), which interprets the compiled Java bytecode.

Key features of Java programming include:

a. Object-Oriented Programming (OOP): Java is built around the concept of objects, which are instances of classes. OOP principles such as encapsulation, inheritance, and polymorphism are fundamental to Java programming.

b. Strong Typing: Java is a strongly-typed language, meaning that variables must be declared with a specific data type, and type conversions must be explicit. This helps catch type-related errors at compile time.

c. Memory Management: Java uses automatic memory management through a garbage collector. The garbage collector automatically frees up memory that is no longer being used by the program, reducing the chances of memory leaks.

d. Exception Handling: Java provides a robust exception handling mechanism to handle runtime errors gracefully. Exceptions can be caught and handled using try-catch blocks, allowing for proper error handling and recovery.

e. Rich Standard Library: Java comes with a comprehensive standard library that provides a wide range of classes and methods for common tasks such as input/output, networking, data structures, and more.

Here's a simple example of a Java program that prints

"Hello, World!" to the console:

```java
public class HelloWorld {
   public static void main(String[] args) {
      System.out.println("Hello, World!");
   }
}
```

In this example, we define a class named HelloWorld with a main method, which serves as the entry point of the program. The main method is declared as public static void, indicating that it is accessible from anywhere, belongs to the class rather than an instance, and does not return a value. Inside the main method, we use System.out.println() to print the string "Hello, World!" to the console.

To compile and run a Java program, you need to have the Java Development Kit (JDK) installed on your system. The JDK includes the Java compiler (javac), which compiles the Java source code into bytecode, and the Java runtime (java), which executes the compiled bytecode.

Here are the steps to compile and run the above program:

1. Save the code in a file named HelloWorld.java.

2. Open a terminal or command prompt and navigate to the directory where the file is saved.

3. Compile the code using the command: javac HelloWorld.java. This will generate a bytecode file named HelloWorld.class.

4. Run the program using the command: java HelloWorld. This will execute the bytecode and display the output "Hello, World!" in the console.

Java's object-oriented nature, extensive libraries, and robustness make it well-suited for developing healthcare software applications. It provides the necessary tools and frameworks for building scalable, secure, and maintainable solutions

11.2 Developing Electronic Health Record Systems

Electronic Health Record (EHR) systems are digital

versions of patients' medical records that store and manage healthcare information. EHR systems play a crucial role in modern healthcare, enabling efficient storage, retrieval, and sharing of patient data among healthcare providers. Java, with its robustness and extensive libraries, is well-suited for developing EHR systems.

Key considerations when developing EHR systems using Java:

1. Data Modeling: Designing an appropriate data model is essential for an EHR system. Java's object-oriented nature allows for creating classes that represent entities such as patients, encounters, medications, and allergies. These classes encapsulate the data and behavior associated with each entity.

2. Database Integration: EHR systems typically store data in a relational database. Java provides libraries like JDBC (Java Database Connectivity) and ORM (Object-Relational Mapping) frameworks like Hibernate for seamless integration with databases. These tools facilitate database operations such as inserting, retrieving, updating, and deleting records.

3. Security and Privacy: Ensuring the security and privacy of patient data is critical in EHR systems. Java offers robust security features, including built-in encryption libraries, secure communication protocols (e.g., HTTPS), and authentication and authorization mechanisms. Implementing role-based access control (RBAC) and adhering to healthcare standards like HIPAA (Health Insurance Portability and Accountability Act) is essential.

4. User Interface Development: Developing a user-friendly and intuitive user interface is crucial for an EHR system. Java provides various UI frameworks, such as JavaFX and Swing, for creating desktop applications. Web-based EHR systems can be developed using Java web frameworks like Spring or JavaServer Faces (JSF) in combination with HTML, CSS, and JavaScript.

5. Interoperability: EHR systems often need to exchange data with other healthcare systems, such as laboratory information systems (LIS) or picture archiving and communication systems (PACS). Java supports standard healthcare data exchange formats like HL7 (Health Level

Seven) and FHIR (Fast Healthcare Interoperability Resources). Libraries like HAPI (HL7 application programming interface) can be used to parse and generate HL7 messages.

Here's an example of a Java class representing a patient in an EHR system:

```java
public class Patient {
    private String patientId;
    private String firstName;
    private String lastName;
    private Date dateOfBirth;
    private String gender;
    // Other patient attributes

    // Constructor
    public Patient(String patientId, String firstName, String lastName, Date dateOfBirth, String gender) {
        this.patientId = patientId;
        this.firstName = firstName;
        this.lastName = lastName;
        this.dateOfBirth = dateOfBirth;
        this.gender = gender;
    }

    // Getters and setters
    // ...
}
```

In this example, the Patient class encapsulates the data associated with a patient, such as the patient ID, name, date of birth, and gender. The constructor allows creating a new patient object with the specified attributes. Getters and setters (not shown) provide access to these attributes.

To persist patient data in a database, you can use JDBC or an ORM framework like Hibernate. Here's an example of saving a patient record using JDBC:

```java
public void savePatient(Patient patient) {
    String sql = "INSERT INTO patients (patient_id, first_name, last_name, date_of_birth, gender) VALUES (?, ?, ?, ?, ?)";
    try (Connection connection = getConnection();
        PreparedStatement statement = connection.prepareStatement(sql)) {
        statement.setString(1, patient.getPatientId());
        statement.setString(2, patient.getFirstName());
```

```
        statement.setString(3, patient.getLastName());
        statement.setDate(4,                           new
    java.sql.Date(patient.getDateOfBirth().getTime()));
        statement.setString(5, patient.getGender());
        statement.executeUpdate();
    } catch (SQLException e) {
        // Handle the exception
    }
}
```

In this example, the savePatient method takes a Patient object and inserts its data into the patients table using a prepared statement. The getConnection() method (not shown) establishes a connection to the database.

Developing an EHR system involves many more components, such as handling medical encounters, prescriptions, allergies, and generating reports. Java's extensive libraries and frameworks provide the necessary tools to build these components efficiently.

When developing an EHR system, it's important to follow best practices for software development, including modular design, unit testing, error handling, and logging. Additionally, compliance with healthcare regulations and standards should be a top priority throughout the development process.

Java's robustness, scalability, and rich ecosystem make it a suitable choice for developing EHR systems. Its object-oriented nature, combined with powerful libraries and frameworks, enables the creation of secure, interoperable, and user-friendly healthcare software solutions

Case Study 1: Building a Medication Tracking App

Objective

In this case study, we will develop a medication tracking app using Java to help patients manage their medication schedules and improve adherence. The app will allow users to input their prescribed medications, set reminders, and track their medication intake.

Features

1. User Registration and Authentication: Users can create an account and log in to the app securely.
2. Medication Management: Users can add, edit, and delete their medications, including details like dosage, frequency, and instructions.
3. Reminder System: Users can set reminders for each medication, specifying the time and frequency of intake. The app will send notifications to remind users to take their medications.
4. Medication Tracking: Users can mark medications as taken or skipped, allowing them to track their medication adherence over time.
5. Reporting and Analytics: The app will generate reports and visualizations of the user's medication adherence, providing insights into their medication-taking habits.

Implementation

1. User Interface: Develop a user-friendly interface using JavaFX or Swing for the desktop app, or use Java web frameworks like Spring or JavaServer Faces (JSF) for a web-based app.
2. Database: Use a relational database like MySQL or PostgreSQL to store user information, medication details, and medication tracking data. Utilize JDBC or an ORM framework like Hibernate for database integration.
3.Authentication and Security: Implement user authentication using techniques like password hashing and secure storage of user credentials. Ensure secure communication between the app and the server using HTTPS.
4.Reminder System: Use Java's built-in scheduling capabilities, such as the java.util.concurrent package or libraries like Quartz, to schedule and trigger medication reminders.
5. Reporting and Analytics: Utilize Java libraries like JFreeChart or Apache POI to generate charts and export data for reporting and analysis.

Conclusion

We can provide patients with a convenient tool to manage their medication schedules, improve adherence, and ultimately contribute to better healthcare outcomes by developing a medication tracking app using Java. The app's features, such as reminders and tracking, empower patients to take control of their medication management and facilitate communication with healthcare providers.

Case Study 2: Developing a Telemedicine Platform

Objective

In this case study, we will develop a telemedicine platform using Java to enable remote consultations between patients and healthcare providers. The platform will facilitate video conferencing, secure messaging, and the exchange of medical information.

Features

1. User Roles: The platform will support different user roles, including patients, healthcare providers, and administrators, each with specific access rights and functionalities.

2.Video Conferencing: Integrate video conferencing capabilities using Java libraries like WebRTC or third-party APIs to enable real-time video consultations between patients and healthcare providers.

3.Secure Messaging: Implement secure messaging functionality, allowing patients and healthcare providers to communicate asynchronously and exchange medical information, such as test results or prescription requests.

4.Electronic Health Records (EHR) Integration: Integrate the platform with an existing EHR system to retrieve and display relevant patient information during consultations.

5.Scheduling and Appointments: Enable patients to schedule appointments with healthcare providers through the platform, considering provider availability and time zones.

6.Security and Privacy: Ensure end-to-end encryption for video consultations and secure storage of patient data in compliance with healthcare regulations like HIPAA.

Implementation

1. Backend Development: Use Java frameworks like Spring Boot or Java EE to develop the backend server, handling user authentication, data storage, and business logic.

2. Frontend Development: Develop the user interface using web technologies like HTML, CSS, and JavaScript, utilizing Java web frameworks like JavaServer Faces (JSF) or Vaadin for server-side rendering.

3. Video Conferencing: Integrate video conferencing functionality using WebRTC libraries like Jitsi Meet or third-party APIs like Twilio or Agora.

4. Secure Messaging: Implement secure messaging using encryption techniques like SSL/TLS for data transmission and secure storage of messages in the database.

5. EHR Integration: Use Java's interoperability features, such as HL7 libraries or FHIR APIs, to integrate with existing EHR systems and retrieve patient data securely.

6. Scheduling and Appointments: Utilize Java libraries like Quartz or jCron for scheduling and managing appointments, considering timezone conversions and provider availability.

Conclusion:

Developing a telemedicine platform using Java enables remote healthcare delivery, improving access to medical services and reducing barriers to care. The platform's features, such as video conferencing, secure messaging, and EHR integration, facilitate effective communication and collaboration between patients and healthcare providers. We can build a scalable and secure telemedicine solution that enhances the quality of healthcare services by utilizing Java's robust libraries and frameworks.

12 C++ PROGRAMMING FOR HIGH-PERFORMANCE COMPUTING IN HEALTHCARE

C++ is a powerful and versatile programming language known for its performance, efficiency, and low-level control. It is widely used in various domains, including healthcare, where high-performance computing is crucial for handling large datasets, complex simulations, and real-time data processing. C++'s ability to deliver fast execution and optimize resource utilization makes it a popular choice for developing high-performance healthcare applications.

12.1 Introduction to C++ Programming

C++ is an extension of the C programming language, adding object-oriented programming (OOP) features and enhanced functionality. It combines the low-level control of C with the high-level abstractions and OOP concepts, making it suitable for both system-level programming and application development.

Key features of C++ programming include:

a. Object-Oriented Programming (OOP): C++ supports OOP principles such as encapsulation, inheritance, and polymorphism. It allows the creation of classes and objects, enabling modular and reusable code design.

b. Performance and Efficiency: C++ is known for its performance and efficiency. It allows low-level memory manipulation, direct hardware access, and fine-grained control over system resources, enabling developers to optimize code for speed and memory usage.

c. Standard Template Library (STL): C++ provides a powerful standard library called the Standard Template Library (STL). The STL offers a collection of reusable components, such as containers (e.g., vectors, lists, maps), algorithms (e.g., sorting, searching), and iterators, which greatly simplify common programming tasks.

d. Generic Programming: C++ supports generic programming through templates. Templates allow the creation of reusable code that can work with different data types, enabling the development of flexible and type-independent algorithms and data structures.

e. Exception Handling: C++ provides a robust exception handling mechanism to handle runtime errors gracefully. Exceptions can be thrown and caught, allowing for proper error handling and recovery in exceptional situations.

Here's a simple example of a C++ program that calculates the body mass index (BMI) based on a person's weight and height:

```cpp
#include <iostream>
using namespace std;

double calculateBMI(double weight, double height) {
    return weight / (height * height);
}

int main() {
    double weight, height;
    cout << "Enter weight (in kilograms): ";
```

```
cin >> weight;
cout << "Enter height (in meters): ";
cin >> height;

double bmi = calculateBMI(weight, height);
cout << "BMI: " << bmi << endl;

return 0;
}
```

In this example, we define a function calculateBMI that takes a person's weight (in kilograms) and height (in meters) as input and returns the calculated BMI. In the main function, we prompt the user to enter their weight and height, call the calculateBMI function, and display the result.

To compile and run a C++ program, you need a C++ compiler installed on your system, such as GCC (GNU Compiler Collection) or Clang. Here are the steps to compile and run the above program using GCC:

1. Save the code in a file named bmi.cpp.

2. Open a terminal or command prompt and navigate to the directory where the file is saved.

3. Compile the code using the command: g++ bmi.cpp -o bmi. This will generate an executable file named bmi.

4. Run the program using the command: ./bmi (on Unix/Linux) or bmi.exe (on Windows). Enter the required inputs and observe the output.

C++'s performance, efficiency, and low-level control make it well-suited for developing high-performance healthcare applications. Its OOP features and generic programming capabilities enable the creation of modular, reusable, and maintainable code

12.2 Optimizing Algorithms for Large-Scale Data Processing

In healthcare, large-scale data processing is often required to analyze vast amounts of patient records, medical images, genomic data, and sensor data.

Optimizing algorithms for efficient processing of such large datasets is crucial to ensure timely insights and decision-making. C++, with its focus on performance and low-level control, provides various techniques and libraries for optimizing algorithms for large-scale data processing.

12.2.1. Algorithmic Optimization

Choose appropriate data structures: Select data structures that are efficient for the specific problem at hand. For example, using hash tables for fast lookups or using priority queues for efficient sorting and searching.

Minimize data copying: Avoid unnecessary data copying by using references or pointers instead of copying objects. This reduces memory usage and improves performance.

Leverage parallelism: Utilize parallel programming techniques, such as multi-threading or distributed computing, to process data in parallel and harness the power of multiple cores or machines.

12.2.2. Memory Management

Allocate and deallocate memory efficiently: Use memory pools or custom allocators to minimize the overhead of frequent memory allocation and deallocation operations.

Optimize memory layout: Arrange data in memory to maximize cache locality and minimize cache misses. This can be achieved through techniques like data structure padding and cache-conscious data layout.

Minimize memory footprint: Reduce the memory usage of algorithms by using compact data representations, such as bit-packing or compression, when appropriate.

12.2.3. Parallel Programming

Utilize multi-threading: Leverage C++'s threading capabilities, such as the std::thread library or libraries like OpenMP, to parallelize computationally intensive tasks and distribute the workload across multiple cores.

Employ SIMD instructions: Utilize Single Instruction, Multiple Data (SIMD) instructions, such as SSE or AVX, to perform parallel operations on multiple data elements simultaneously, improving the efficiency of data-parallel computations.

Harness GPU acceleration: Utilize GPU programming frameworks like CUDA or OpenCL to offload computationally intensive tasks to the GPU, utilizing its massive parallel processing capabilities.

12.2.4. Profiling and Optimization:

Profile the code: Use profiling tools to identify performance bottlenecks, such as hotspots or memory leaks, and focus

optimization efforts on critical sections of the code.

Optimize algorithms: Apply algorithmic optimizations, such as reducing the time complexity, minimizing iterations, or using efficient search techniques, to improve the performance of critical algorithms.

Optimize compilers: Utilize compiler optimizations, such as enabling higher optimization levels (-O2 or -O3) or using profile-guided optimization (PGO), to let the compiler make informed optimizations based on runtime behavior.

Here's an example of optimizing a simple algorithm for calculating the sum of a large array using parallel programming with OpenMP:

```cpp
#include <iostream>
#include <vector>
#include <omp.h>

long long parallelSum(const std::vector<int>& arr) {
    long long sum = 0;
    #pragma omp parallel for reduction(+:sum)
    for (int i = 0; i < arr.size(); ++i) {
        sum += arr[i];
    }
    return sum;
}

int main() {
    std::vector<int> largeArray(100000000, 1);
```

```cpp
        double start = omp_get_wtime();
        long long sum = parallelSum(largeArray);
        double end = omp_get_wtime();

        std::cout << "Sum: " << sum << std::endl;
        std::cout << "Execution time: " << (end - start) << " seconds"
    << std::endl;

        return 0;
    }
```

In this example, the parallelSum function calculates the sum of a large array using OpenMP's parallel for loop. The #pragma omp parallel for directive instructs the compiler to distribute the loop iterations among multiple threads. The reduction(+:sum) clause ensures that the partial sums calculated by each thread are correctly combined into the final sum.

The computation is distributed across multiple cores, significantly reducing the execution time compared to a sequential implementation by utilizing parallel programming.

Optimizing algorithms for large-scale data processing in healthcare requires a combination of algorithmic optimization, memory management, parallel programming, and profiling techniques. C++, with its performance-focused features and extensive libraries, provides the necessary tools and capabilities to develop efficient and scalable algorithms for processing large datasets in healthcare applications.

It's important to note that optimization is an iterative process, and the specific optimizations applied depend on the nature of the problem, the hardware architecture, and the performance requirements. Profiling and benchmarking are essential to identify performance bottlenecks and measure the effectiveness of optimizations

Case Study 1: Accelerating Drug Discovery with Parallel Computing

Objective

In this case study, we will explore how C++ and parallel computing techniques can be used to accelerate the drug discovery process. Drug discovery involves screening large libraries of chemical compounds to identify potential drug candidates. We can significantly reduce the time required for virtual screening and molecular simulations, enabling faster identification of promising drug leads by utilizing parallel computing.

Problem

Virtual screening is a computationally intensive process that involves evaluating the binding affinity of a large number of chemical compounds against a specific drug target. The goal is to identify compounds that show promising interaction with the target and have the potential to become effective drugs. However, the sheer size of chemical libraries and the complexity of molecular simulations make this process time-consuming when performed sequentially.

Solution

To accelerate the drug discovery process, we can harness the power of parallel computing using C++. We can significantly reduce the time required for virtual screening and molecular simulations by distributing the computational workload across multiple cores or nodes. Here's a high-level approach:

1. Data Parallelism:

a. Partition the chemical library into smaller subsets that can be processed independently.
b. Assign each subset to a different processor or core for parallel execution.
c. Utilize C++'s threading capabilities, such as the std::thread library or OpenMP, to distribute the workload among multiple threads.

2. Molecular Docking:

a. Implement or integrate a molecular docking algorithm, such as AutoDock or GOLD, to evaluate the binding affinity between the chemical compounds and the drug target.

b. Parallelize the docking calculations by running multiple instances of the docking algorithm concurrently on different subsets of the chemical library.

c. Utilize C++'s low-level control and performance optimizations to minimize the overhead of parallel execution.

3. Molecular Dynamics Simulations:

a. Perform molecular dynamics simulations to assess the stability and dynamics of the protein-ligand complexes.

b. Utilize high-performance molecular dynamics libraries, such as GROMACS or OpenMM, which are optimized for parallel execution.

c. Distribute the simulation workload across multiple nodes or GPUs to leverage their parallel processing capabilities.

4. Result Aggregation and Analysis:

a. Collect and aggregate the results from parallel computations, such as docking scores and simulation trajectories.

b. Perform post-processing and analysis on the aggregated data to identify the most promising drug candidates.

c. Utilize C++'s efficient data structures and algorithms to handle large datasets and perform complex analysis tasks.

Example:

Here's a simplified example of parallel virtual screening using OpenMP in C++:

```cpp
#include <iostream>
#include <vector>
#include <omp.h>

struct Compound {
    // Compound properties
};

double calculateBindingAffinity(const Compound& compound)
{
```

```cpp
  // Perform docking calculations and return binding affinity
}

std::vector<Compound>                    screenCompounds(const
std::vector<Compound>& library, double affinityThreshold) {
   std::vector<Compound> hits;
   #pragma omp parallel for
   for (int i = 0; i < library.size(); ++i) {
      double affinity = calculateBindingAffinity(library[i]);
      if (affinity >= affinityThreshold) {
         #pragma omp critical
         {
            hits.push_back(library[i]);
         }
      }
   }
    return hits;
}

int main() {
   std::vector<Compound> chemicalLibrary = // Load chemical
library
   double affinityThreshold = // Set affinity threshold

   std::vector<Compound>          drugCandidates          =
screenCompounds(chemicalLibrary, affinityThreshold);

   // Process and analyze drug candidates

   return 0;
}
```

In this example, the screenCompounds function performs parallel virtual screening on a chemical library. The #pragma omp parallel for directive distributes the loop iterations among multiple threads, allowing each thread to calculate the binding affinity of a subset of compounds independently. Compounds with binding affinities above the specified threshold are collected as potential drug candidates using a critical section to ensure thread safety.

The virtual screening process can be significantly accelerated, enabling faster identification of promising drug candidates by using parallel computing. The actual implementation would involve more complex docking algorithms, molecular dynamics simulations, and result analysis, but the principle of parallel execution remains the same.

Conclusion

Parallel computing, combined with the performance and low-level control of C++, offers a powerful approach to accelerate the drug discovery process. We can significantly reduce the time required for virtual screening and molecular simulations by distributing the computational workload across multiple cores or nodes. This enables faster identification of promising drug candidates, ultimately accelerating the development of new medicines.

Parallel computing in drug discovery is not limited to virtual screening; it can also be applied to other computationally intensive tasks, such as protein folding simulations, pharmacokinetic modeling, and ADME (Absorption, Distribution, Metabolism, and Excretion) predictions. With the power of parallel computing and C++'s performance optimizations, researchers can tackle complex computational challenges and accelerate the pace of drug discovery, bringing new and effective treatments to patients faster.

It's important to note that parallel computing in drug discovery requires careful design, load balancing, and synchronization to ensure correct and efficient execution. Proper benchmarking, profiling, and optimization are essential to achieve optimal performance and scalability

Case Study 2: Accelerating Medical Image Analysis with GPU Computing

Objective

In this case study, we will explore how C++ and GPU computing can be used to accelerate medical image analysis tasks, such as image segmentation and feature extraction. Medical imaging, including CT scans, MRI, and PET scans, generates large volumes of high-resolution images that require extensive processing. The parallel processing capabilities of GPUs can significantly reduce the time required for image analysis, enabling faster diagnosis and treatment planning.

Problem

Medical image analysis involves computationally intensive tasks, such as image segmentation, which aims to identify and delineate specific anatomical structures or regions of interest in medical images. These tasks often require processing large datasets of high-resolution images, which can be time-consuming when performed on traditional CPUs. The goal is to accelerate these tasks to improve the efficiency and speed of medical image analysis workflows.

Solution

To accelerate medical image analysis, we can harness the power of GPU computing using C++ and CUDA (Compute Unified Device Architecture). CUDA is a parallel computing platform and programming model developed by NVIDIA for general computing on GPUs.

Here's a high-level approach:

1. Image Data Transfer

Transfer the medical image data from the CPU memory to the GPU memory efficiently using CUDA's memory transfer functions.

Utilize CUDA streams to overlap data transfer with computation, minimizing idle time and maximizing GPU utilization.

2. Parallel Image Segmentation:

Implement image segmentation algorithms, such as thresholding or region growing, using CUDA kernels.

Partition the image into smaller tiles or blocks that can be processed independently by different GPU threads.

Leverage CUDA's parallel execution model to perform segmentation calculations simultaneously on multiple pixels or regions of the image.

3. Feature Extraction:

Implement feature extraction algorithms, such as edge detection or texture analysis, using CUDA kernels.

Parallelize the feature extraction calculations by distributing the workload across GPU threads.

Utilize CUDA's shared memory and memory coalescing techniques to optimize memory access patterns and minimize latency.

4. Result Visualization and Analysis:

Transfer the processed image data and extracted features back from the GPU memory to the CPU memory.

Visualize the segmented images and extracted features using appropriate libraries or frameworks, such as OpenCV or VTK.

Perform further analysis or downstream processing on the extracted features for diagnosis or treatment planning.

Example:
Here's a simplified example of parallel image thresholding using CUDA in C++:

```cpp
#include <iostream>
#include <vector>
#include <cuda_runtime.h>

__global__ void thresholdKernel(unsigned char* image, int width, int height, unsigned char threshold) {
    int x = blockIdx.x * blockDim.x + threadIdx.x;
    int y = blockIdx.y * blockDim.y + threadIdx.y;

    if (x < width && y < height) {
        int index = y * width + x;
        image[index] = (image[index] > threshold) ? 255 : 0;
    }
}

void thresholdImage(std::vector<unsigned char>& image, int width, int height, unsigned char threshold) {
    unsigned char* deviceImage;
    cudaMalloc(&deviceImage, image.size() * sizeof(unsigned char));
    cudaMemcpy(deviceImage, image.data(), image.size() * sizeof(unsigned char), cudaMemcpyHostToDevice);
```

```
    dim3 blockSize(16, 16);
    dim3 gridSize((width + blockSize.x - 1) / blockSize.x, (height
+ blockSize.y - 1) / blockSize.y);

    thresholdKernel<<<gridSize,        blockSize>>>(deviceImage,
    width, height, threshold);

    cudaMemcpy(image.data(),    deviceImage,    image.size()    *
    sizeof(unsigned char), cudaMemcpyDeviceToHost);
        cudaFree(deviceImage);
    }

    int main() {
    std::vector<unsigned char> medicalImage = // Load medical
    image data
        int width = // Image width
        int height = // Image height
        unsigned char threshold = // Segmentation threshold

    thresholdImage(medicalImage, width, height, threshold);

        // Visualize and analyze the segmented image

        return 0;
    }
```

In this example, the thresholdKernel function is a CUDA kernel that performs parallel image thresholding. Each GPU thread processes a single pixel of the image, comparing its intensity value against the specified threshold. Pixels with intensities above the threshold are set to white (255), while others are set to black (0).

The thresholdImage function allocates memory on the GPU, transfers the image data from the CPU to the GPU, launches the CUDA kernel with appropriate block and grid sizes, and transfers the processed image data back to the CPU.

GPU computing can significantly accelerate the image thresholding operation compared to sequential execution on a CPU. The same principle can be applied to more complex image segmentation and feature extraction algorithms, enabling faster processing of large medical image datasets.

Conclusion

GPU computing, combined with the performance and low-level control of C++, offers a powerful approach to accelerate medical image analysis tasks. The parallel processing capabilities of GPUs can significantly reduce the time required for image segmentation, feature extraction, and other computationally intensive operations. This enables faster diagnosis, treatment planning, and overall improvement in the efficiency of medical imaging workflows.

GPU computing in medical image analysis is not limited to image segmentation; it can also be applied to other tasks, such as image registration, 3D reconstruction, and machine learning-based image classification. Healthcare professionals can process and analyze medical images more efficiently through the power of GPU computing and C++'s performance optimizations, leading to better patient care and outcomes.

It's important to note that GPU computing requires careful consideration of data transfer overhead, memory management, and kernel optimization to achieve optimal performance. Proper profiling, debugging, and performance tuning are essential to ensure efficient utilization of GPU resources and maximize the benefits of parallel processing.

In conclusion, C++ and GPU computing technologies offer immense potential in accelerating medical image analysis tasks, enabling faster and more efficient processing of large medical image datasets. Healthcare professionals can expedite the diagnosis and treatment planning process, ultimately improving patient care and outcomes by utilizing the power of parallel computing.

Case Study 3: Optimizing Genomic Data Analysis with Distributed Computing

Objective

In this case study, we will explore how C++ and distributed computing techniques can be used to optimize genomic data analysis workflows. Genomic data, such as DNA sequencing data, is characterized by its massive size and complexity. Analyzing and processing genomic data often requires substantial computational resources and time. We can distribute the workload across multiple nodes or clusters, enabling faster and more efficient analysis of genomic datasets by using distributed computing.

Problem

Genomic data analysis involves various computationally intensive tasks, such as sequence alignment, variant calling, and genome assembly. These tasks often require processing terabytes or even petabytes of data, which can be time-consuming and resource-intensive when performed on a single machine. The goal is to optimize these workflows by distributing the computational workload across multiple nodes, enabling parallel processing and reducing the overall analysis time.

Solution

To optimize genomic data analysis workflows, we can leverage distributed computing frameworks and C++'s performance optimizations. Here's a high-level approach:
1. Data Partitioning and Distribution:
    a. Partition the genomic dataset into smaller chunks that can be processed independently.
    b. Distribute the partitioned data across multiple nodes in a cluster or distributed computing environment.
    c. Utilize distributed file systems, such as Hadoop
    d. Distributed File System (HDFS) or Lustre, to efficiently store and access the partitioned data.

2. Parallel Sequence Alignment:

Implement parallel sequence alignment algorithms, such as Burrows-Wheeler Aligner (BWA) or Bowtie, using C++ and distributed computing frameworks like Apache Spark or MPI (Message Passing Interface).

Distribute the alignment tasks across multiple nodes, allowing each node to process a subset of the genomic data in parallel.

Utilize C++'s low-level optimizations and efficient data structures to minimize the overhead of parallel execution and maximize performance.

3. Distributed Variant Calling:

Perform variant calling on the aligned sequences using distributed computing frameworks like Apache Spark or GATK (Genome Analysis Toolkit).

Parallelize the variant calling process by distributing the workload across multiple nodes, enabling faster identification of genetic variations.

Leverage C++'s performance optimizations and efficient algorithms to speed up the variant calling calculations.

4. Genome Assembly and Analysis:

Implement distributed genome assembly algorithms, such as de Bruijn graph-based assemblers, using C++ and distributed computing frameworks.

Distribute the assembly tasks across multiple nodes, allowing parallel construction of the genome from the sequenced fragments.

Perform downstream analysis, such as annotation and functional analysis, on the assembled genome using distributed computing techniques.

Example:

Here's a simplified example of parallel sequence alignment using Apache Spark and C++:

```cpp
#include <iostream>
#include <vector>
```

```cpp
#include <spark/spark.h>

void alignSequences(const std::vector<std::string>& sequences,
const std::string& reference) {
    // Implement sequence alignment algorithm (e.g., BWA or
Bowtie)
    // Align each sequence against the reference genome
    // Return the aligned sequences
}

int main() {
    // Initialize Spark context
    spark::SparkContext sc;

    // Load genomic sequences from distributed file system (e.g.,
HDFS)
    auto sequences = sc.textFile("hdfs://path/to/sequences");

    // Load reference genome
    std::string referenceGenome = // Load reference genome data

    // Distribute sequence alignment tasks across Spark nodes
    auto    alignedSequences    =    sequences.map([&](const
std::string& sequence) {
        return alignSequences({sequence}, referenceGenome);
    });

    // Collect aligned sequences
    std::vector<std::string>            alignments            =
alignedSequences.collect();

    // Perform further analysis on the aligned sequences

    return 0;
}
```

In this example, we use Apache Spark, a distributed computing framework, to parallelize the sequence alignment process. The genomic sequences are loaded from a distributed file system (e.g., HDFS) into an RDD (Resilient Distributed Dataset) in Spark.

The alignSequences function represents the sequence alignment algorithm (e.g., BWA or Bowtie) implemented in C++. It aligns each sequence against the reference genome and returns the aligned sequences.

The map operation in Spark distributes the alignment tasks across multiple nodes in the Spark cluster. Each node independently aligns a subset of the sequences against the reference genome using the alignSequences function.

Finally, the aligned sequences are collected back to the driver program for further analysis.

We can significantly accelerate genomic data analysis workflows by employing distributed computing frameworks like Apache Spark and C++'s performance optimizations. The workload is distributed across multiple nodes, enabling parallel processing and reducing the overall analysis time.

Conclusion

Distributed computing, combined with the performance and low-level control of C++, offers a powerful approach to optimize genomic data analysis workflows. We can significantly reduce the time required for sequence alignment, variant calling, genome assembly, and other computationally intensive tasks by distributing the computational workload across multiple nodes or clusters. This enables faster and more efficient analysis of large genomic datasets, accelerating research and clinical applications.

Distributed computing in genomic data analysis is not limited to the examples mentioned above; it can be applied to various other tasks, such as phylogenetic analysis, gene expression analysis, and genomic data compression. Researchers and healthcare professionals can process and analyze genomic data more efficiently, leading to faster discoveries and advancements in genomic medicine by harnessing the power of distributed computing and C++'s performance optimizations.

It's important to note that distributed computing requires careful design, data partitioning, and load balancing to ensure optimal performance and scalability. Proper configuration, monitoring, and optimization of the distributed computing environment are essential to maximize resource utilization and minimize overhead.

13 DATABASE MANAGEMENT WITH SQL IN HEALTHCARE

13.1 Introduction to SQL and Relational Databases
In the healthcare industry, efficient management and retrieval of data are crucial for various purposes, such as patient care, medical research, and administrative tasks. Structured Query Language (SQL) and relational databases provide a powerful framework for storing, organizing, and accessing healthcare data in a structured and efficient manner.

13.2 Understanding SQL and Relational Databases
SQL is a standardized language used for managing and manipulating relational databases. It allows users to create, modify, and query databases using a set of predefined commands and statements. SQL is widely used in healthcare due to its simplicity, flexibility, and ability to handle large volumes of structured data.

Relational databases, on the other hand, are based on the relational model, which organizes data into tables consisting of rows (records) and columns (fields). Each table represents a specific entity or concept, such as patients, medications, or diagnoses. Tables are related to each other through common fields, enabling the establishment of relationships and the retrieval of data across multiple tables.

13.2 Key concepts in SQL and Relational Databases
1. Tables: Tables are the fundamental building blocks of a relational database. They consist of rows and columns, where each row represents a unique record and each column represents a specific attribute or field.

2. Primary Key: A primary key is a unique identifier for each record in a table. It ensures the uniqueness and integrity of the data and is often used to establish

relationships between tables.

3. Foreign Key: A foreign key is a field in one table that refers to the primary key of another table. It establishes a relationship between two tables, enabling the retrieval of related data across multiple tables.

4. SQL Statements: SQL provides a set of statements for interacting with databases, including:

a. SELECT: Used to retrieve data from one or more tables based on specified criteria.

b. INSERT: Used to insert new records into a table.

c. UPDATE: Used to modify existing records in a table.

d. DELETE: Used to delete records from a table.

e. CREATE: Used to create new tables, indexes, or other database objects.

f. ALTER: Used to modify the structure of existing tables or other database objects.

Benefits of Using SQL and Relational Databases in Healthcare:

Data Integrity: SQL and relational databases enforce data integrity through constraints, such as primary keys and foreign keys, ensuring the accuracy and consistency of healthcare data.

Data Retrieval: SQL provides powerful querying capabilities, allowing healthcare professionals to retrieve specific subsets of data based on various criteria, such as patient demographics, diagnoses, or treatment outcomes.

Data Analysis: SQL enables complex data analysis by allowing the combination and aggregation of data from multiple tables. This facilitates tasks such as identifying trends, generating reports, and supporting clinical decision-making.

Data Security: SQL and relational databases offer built-in security features, such as user authentication, access control, and data encryption, ensuring the confidentiality and protection of sensitive healthcare information.

Scalability: Relational databases can handle large volumes of data and can scale to accommodate the growing needs of healthcare organizations. They provide efficient storage and retrieval mechanisms, even for massive datasets.

Example:
Let's consider a simplified example of a healthcare database schema:

```sql
-- Patients Table
CREATE TABLE Patients (
  PatientID INT PRIMARY KEY,
  FirstName VARCHAR(50),
  LastName VARCHAR(50),
  DateOfBirth DATE,
  Gender VARCHAR(10)
);

-- Diagnoses Table
CREATE TABLE Diagnoses (
  DiagnosisID INT PRIMARY KEY,
  PatientID INT,
  DiagnosisCode VARCHAR(10),
  DiagnosisDate DATE,
  FOREIGN KEY (PatientID) REFERENCES Patients(PatientID)
);
```

In this example, we have two tables: Patients and Diagnoses. The Patients table stores basic patient information, such as name, date of birth, and gender. The Diagnoses table stores information about the diagnoses associated with each patient, including the diagnosis code and date.

The PatientID field in the Patients table serves as the primary key, uniquely identifying each patient record. The PatientID field in the Diagnoses table is a foreign key that references the PatientID in the Patients table, establishing a relationship between the two tables.

To retrieve the diagnoses for a specific patient, we can use an SQL query like:

```sql
SELECT p.FirstName, p.LastName, d.DiagnosisCode, d.DiagnosisDate
FROM Patients p
```

```
JOIN Diagnoses d ON p.PatientID = d.PatientID
WHERE p.PatientID = 1;
```

This query joins the Patients and Diagnoses tables based on the PatientID field and retrieves the first name, last name, diagnosis code, and diagnosis date for the patient with PatientID equal to 1.

SQL and relational databases provide a structured and efficient way to manage and analyze healthcare data. Healthcare organizations can store, retrieve, and manipulate data effectively, enabling better patient care, research, and decision-making by utilizing the power of SQL.

Understanding the fundamentals of SQL and relational databases is essential for healthcare professionals and data analysts working with healthcare data. It allows them to design and implement robust database schemas, perform complex queries, and extract meaningful insights from the data.

13.3 Querying and Managing Electronic Health Records

Electronic Health Records (EHRs) have revolutionized the way patient data is stored, accessed, and utilized in healthcare. EHRs provide a centralized repository for patient information, including demographics, medical history, medications, laboratory results, and clinical notes. SQL plays a crucial role in querying and managing EHRs, enabling healthcare professionals to retrieve and analyze patient data efficiently.

13.3.1 Querying EHRs with SQL

SQL provides a powerful set of commands and clauses for querying EHRs and retrieving specific subsets of patient data. Some common querying techniques include:

SELECT Statement: The SELECT statement is used to retrieve data from one or more tables in the EHR database. It allows you to specify the columns to retrieve, apply filters using the WHERE clause, and sort the results using the ORDER BY clause.

Example:

```
SELECT PatientID, FirstName, LastName, DateOfBirth
FROM Patients
WHERE Gender = 'Female'
ORDER BY LastName;
```

13.3.2 JOIN Operations

SQL supports various types of join operations, such as INNER JOIN, LEFT JOIN, and RIGHT JOIN, which allow you to combine data from multiple tables based on related columns. Joins are essential for retrieving data that spans across different tables in the EHR database.

Example:

```
SELECT        p.PatientID,        p.FirstName,        p.LastName,
d.DiagnosisCode, d.DiagnosisDate
FROM Patients p
INNER JOIN Diagnoses d ON p.PatientID = d.PatientID;
```

13.3.3 Aggregation Functions

SQL provides aggregation functions like COUNT, SUM, AVG, MIN, and MAX, which allow you to perform calculations and summarize data across multiple records. These functions are useful for generating reports and statistical analysis.

Example:

```
SELECT          COUNT(*)          AS          TotalPatients,
AVG(DATEDIFF(YEAR,   DateOfBirth,   GETDATE()))   AS
AvgAge
FROM Patients;
```

13.3.4 Managing EHRs with SQL

In addition to querying, SQL provides statements for managing and manipulating data in EHRs. Some common management tasks include:

Inserting Records: The INSERT statement is used to add new records to a table in the EHR database. It allows you

to specify the values for each column in the new record.
Example:
    INSERT INTO Patients (PatientID, FirstName, LastName, DateOfBirth, Gender)
    VALUES (1, 'John', 'Doe', '1990-05-15', 'Male');
Updating Records: The UPDATE statement is used to modify existing records in a table. It allows you to change the values of specific columns based on specified conditions.

Example:
    UPDATE Patients
    SET LastName = 'Smith'
    WHERE PatientID = 1;
Deleting Records: The DELETE statement is used to remove records from a table based on specified conditions.

Example:
    DELETE FROM Diagnoses
    WHERE PatientID = 1;
Creating and Modifying Tables: SQL provides statements like CREATE TABLE and ALTER TABLE to create new tables and modify the structure of existing tables in the EHR database.

Example:
    CREATE TABLE Medications (
      MedicationID INT PRIMARY KEY,
      PatientID INT,
      MedicationName VARCHAR(100),
      Dosage VARCHAR(50),
      FOREIGN KEY (PatientID) REFERENCES Patients(PatientID)
    );
Healthcare professionals can efficiently retrieve patient data, generate reports, and perform data analysis to support clinical decision-making and improve patient care by utilizing SQL for querying and managing EHRs.

13.4 Case Study: Implementing a Clinical Decision Support System

Clinical Decision Support Systems (CDSS) are computer-based systems that assist healthcare professionals in making clinical decisions by providing relevant information, alerts, and recommendations based on patient data. In this case study, we will explore how SQL and relational databases can be used to implement a CDSS for managing patients with chronic diseases.

Objective

The objective of this case study is to design and implement a CDSS that helps healthcare providers monitor and manage patients with chronic diseases, such as diabetes or hypertension. The system will use SQL and a relational database to store patient data, medical guidelines, and generate alerts and recommendations based on predefined rules.

Database Design

The first step is to design the database schema for the CDSS. The schema should include tables for storing patient information, medical conditions, medications, and clinical guidelines. Here's a simplified example of the database schema:

```
-- Patients Table
CREATE TABLE Patients (
  PatientID INT PRIMARY KEY,
  FirstName VARCHAR(50),
  LastName VARCHAR(50),
  DateOfBirth DATE,
  Gender VARCHAR(10)
);

-- Conditions Table
CREATE TABLE Conditions (
  ConditionID INT PRIMARY KEY,
  PatientID INT,
  ConditionName VARCHAR(100),
  DiagnosisDate DATE,
  FOREIGN KEY (PatientID) REFERENCES Patients(PatientID)
);

-- Medications Table
```

```
CREATE TABLE Medications (
  MedicationID INT PRIMARY KEY,
  PatientID INT,
  MedicationName VARCHAR(100),
  Dosage VARCHAR(50),
  StartDate DATE,
  EndDate DATE,
FOREIGN KEY (PatientID) REFERENCES Patients(PatientID)
);

-- Guidelines Table
CREATE TABLE Guidelines (
  GuidelineID INT PRIMARY KEY,
  ConditionName VARCHAR(100),
  Recommendation VARCHAR(500)
);
```

Querying and Decision Support

Once the database is set up, SQL queries can be used to retrieve patient data and generate alerts and recommendations based on predefined rules. Here are a few examples:

Identifying Patients with Uncontrolled Diabetes

```
SELECT p.PatientID, p.FirstName, p.LastName
FROM Patients p
INNER JOIN Conditions c ON p.PatientID = c.PatientID
WHERE c.ConditionName = 'Diabetes' AND
  NOT EXISTS (
    SELECT *
    FROM Medications m
    WHERE m.PatientID = p.PatientID AND
      m.MedicationName LIKE '%insulin%'
  );
```

This query retrieves the patient information for individuals diagnosed with diabetes who are not currently prescribed insulin. The CDSS can use this information to generate an alert for healthcare providers to review and consider appropriate treatment options.

Providing Medication Recommendations

```
SELECT g.Recommendation
FROM Guidelines g
```

```
WHERE g.ConditionName = 'Hypertension' AND
    g.Recommendation LIKE '%ACE inhibitor%';
```

This query retrieves the medication recommendations from the guidelines table for the management of hypertension, specifically recommending the use of ACE inhibitors. The CDSS can present this recommendation to healthcare providers when they are prescribing medications for patients with hypertension.

Monitoring Medication Adherence:
```
SELECT      p.PatientID,      p.FirstName,      p.LastName,
m.MedicationName, m.EndDate
FROM Patients p
INNER JOIN Medications m ON p.PatientID = m.PatientID
WHERE m.EndDate < GETDATE();
```

This query identifies patients whose medication prescriptions have expired. The CDSS can use this information to generate alerts for healthcare providers to follow up with patients and ensure medication adherence.

The CDSS can provide real-time decision support, alerts, and recommendations to healthcare providers based on patient data and predefined clinical guidelines by utilizing SQL queries and the relational database.

Conclusion

Implementing a Clinical Decision Support System using SQL and relational databases demonstrates the power and flexibility of these technologies in healthcare. Healthcare organizations can create systems that assist in clinical decision-making, improve patient care, and optimize the management of chronic diseases by designing an appropriate database schema and utilizing SQL queries.

The CDSS can be further enhanced by incorporating more complex rules, integrating with external data sources, and providing user-friendly interfaces for healthcare professionals to interact with the system.

14 MATLAB FOR MEDICAL IMAGE

PROCESSING AND SIGNAL ANALYSIS

14.1 Introduction to MATLAB Programming

MATLAB (MATrix LABoratory) is a high-level programming language and numerical computing environment widely used in various fields, including medical image processing and signal analysis. It provides a rich set of built-in functions and toolboxes specifically designed for scientific computing, data visualization, and algorithm development. In this section, we will introduce the basics of MATLAB programming and its application in medical image processing and signal analysis.

Getting Started

To begin using MATLAB, you need to have the MATLAB software installed on your computer. Once installed, you can launch the MATLAB environment and start programming.

The MATLAB user interface consists of several main components:

1. Command Window: This is where you enter MATLAB commands and see the output.

2. Workspace: It displays the variables and their values currently in memory.

3. Current Folder: It shows the files and folders in the current working directory.

4. Editor: It is used for creating and editing MATLAB scripts and functions.

14.2 Basic MATLAB Syntax

MATLAB uses a simple and intuitive syntax for programming. Here are some key elements of the MATLAB syntax:

1. Variables: Variables are used to store data in MATLAB. They are defined using the assignment operator "=". For example:

```
x = 10;
y = [1, 2, 3];
z = 'Hello';
```

2. Matrices and Arrays: MATLAB is designed to work efficiently with matrices and arrays. You can create matrices using square brackets "[]". For example:

```
A = [1, 2, 3; 4, 5, 6; 7, 8, 9];
B = [1:5]; % Creates a row vector [1, 2, 3, 4, 5]
```

3. Operators: MATLAB supports various mathematical operators, such as addition (+), subtraction (-), multiplication (), division (/), and element-wise operations (.). For example:

```
result = A * B'; % Matrix multiplication
element_wise_result = A .* B; % Element-wise multiplication
```

4. Functions: MATLAB provides a wide range of built-in functions for mathematical computations, data analysis, and visualization. You can also create your own custom functions. For example:

```
result = sin(pi/2); % Using the built-in sin function
custom_function = @(x) x^2 + 2*x + 1; % Creating a custom function
```

5. Control Flow: MATLAB supports control flow statements like if-else, for loops, and while loops. These statements allow you to control the execution flow of your program based on certain conditions or iterations.

14.3 Medical Image Processing with MATLAB

MATLAB provides a comprehensive set of tools and functions for medical image processing. The Image Processing Toolbox in MATLAB offers a wide range of algorithms and techniques for image enhancement, segmentation, registration, and analysis. Here are a few examples:

1. Reading and Displaying Medical Images

```
I = imread('brain_mri.jpg'); % Read an MRI image
imshow(I); % Display the image
```

2. Image Enhancement:
```
enhanced_image = imadjust(I); % Adjust image contrast
filtered_image = medfilt2(I); % Apply median filtering for noise
reduction
```

3. Image Segmentation:
```
threshold = graythresh(I); % Compute optimal threshold using
Otsu's method
segmented_image = imbinarize(I, threshold); % Perform binary
segmentation
```

4. Image Registration:
```
fixed_image = imread('fixed_image.jpg');
moving_image = imread('moving_image.jpg');
[optimizer, metric] = imregconfig('multimodal');
moving_reg = imregister(moving_image, fixed_image, 'affine',
optimizer, metric);
```

14.4 Signal Analysis with MATLAB

MATLAB also provides powerful tools for signal analysis, including the Signal Processing Toolbox. It offers functions for signal filtering, frequency analysis, feature extraction, and more. Here are a few examples:

1. Loading and Plotting Signals
```
load('ecg_signal.mat'); % Load an ECG signal from a file
plot(ecg_signal); % Plot the ECG signal
```

2. Signal Filtering
```
fs = 1000; % Sampling frequency
fc = 50; % Cutoff frequency
[b, a] = butter(4, fc/(fs/2)); % Design a Butterworth filter
filtered_signal = filtfilt(b, a, ecg_signal); % Apply the filter
```

3. Frequency Analysis
```
L = length(ecg_signal);
f = fs*(0:(L/2))/L;
Y = fft(ecg_signal);
P2 = abs(Y/L);
P1 = P2(1:L/2+1);
P1(2:end-1) = 2*P1(2:end-1);
plot(f, P1); % Plot the frequency spectrum
```

4. Feature Extraction

features = extractFeatures(ecg_signal); % Extract features from the ECG signal

MATLAB provides a rich set of functions and toolboxes for medical image processing and signal analysis. It allows researchers and practitioners to develop algorithms, analyze data, and visualize results efficiently.

Learning MATLAB programming and exploring its capabilities in medical image processing and signal analysis can greatly enhance your ability to work with medical data and develop innovative solutions in healthcare

14.5 Image Processing Techniques and Toolboxes

MATLAB provides a comprehensive set of image processing techniques and toolboxes that enable users to perform various operations on medical images. These techniques and toolboxes offer a wide range of functionalities for image enhancement, segmentation, registration, and analysis. Let's explore some of the key image processing techniques and toolboxes available in MATLAB.

14.5.1 Image Enhancement Techniques

Image enhancement techniques aim to improve the quality and visual appearance of medical images. MATLAB provides several functions for image enhancement, including:

1. Contrast Adjustment

imadjust: Adjusts the contrast of an image by mapping the intensity values to a new range.

histeq: Performs histogram equalization to enhance the contrast of an image.

2. Noise Reduction

medfilt2: Applies median filtering to reduce salt-and-pepper noise in an image.

wiener2: Performs adaptive noise removal using the Wiener filter.

3.Sharpening

imsharpen: Sharpens an image using unsharp masking or a specified filter.

fspecial and imfilter: Create and apply custom filters for image sharpening.

14.5.2 Image Segmentation Techniques

Image segmentation involves partitioning an image into multiple segments or regions of interest. MATLAB offers various segmentation techniques, such as:

1.Thresholding

graythresh: Computes the optimal threshold value using Otsu's method.

imbinarize: Converts an image to a binary image based on a specified threshold.

2. Edge Detection

edge: Detects edges in an image using various methods like Sobel, Canny, or Prewitt.

imgradient: Computes the gradient magnitude and direction of an image.

3. Region-Based Segmentation

bwlabel: Labels connected components in a binary image.

regionprops: Measures properties of labeled regions, such as area, centroid, or bounding box.

4. Watershed Segmentation

watershed: Performs watershed segmentation on a grayscale image.

imimposemin: Imposes minima at specified locations for marker-controlled watershed segmentation.

14.5.3 Image Registration Techniques

Image registration involves aligning two or more images of the same scene taken at different times, from different viewpoints, or using different imaging modalities. MATLAB provides functions for image registration, including:

1. Intensity-Based Registration

imregister: Registers two images using an optimization algorithm and a similarity metric.

imregtform: Computes the geometric transformation that aligns two images.

2. Feature-Based Registration

detectSURFFeatures and extractFeatures: Detect and extract features from images.

matchFeatures: Matches features between two images.

estimateGeometricTransform: Estimates the geometric transformation between matched features.

14.5.4 Image Processing Toolboxes

MATLAB offers several toolboxes specifically designed for image processing tasks. These toolboxes provide additional functions and algorithms for advanced image analysis. Some notable toolboxes include:

1. Image Processing Toolbox

Provides a wide range of functions for image enhancement, segmentation, registration, and analysis.

Includes tools for image filtering, morphological operations, and color image processing.

2. Computer Vision Toolbox

Offers algorithms for object detection, tracking, and recognition.

Provides functions for feature extraction, stereo vision, and 3D reconstruction.

3. Medical Imaging Toolbox

Provides functions and algorithms specifically designed for medical image analysis.

Includes tools for DICOM file handling, volume visualization, and image registration.

These toolboxes extend the capabilities of MATLAB

for image processing and provide specialized functions for various medical imaging applications.

14.6 Case Study 1: Analyzing ECG Signals

In this case study, we will explore how MATLAB can be used to analyze electrocardiogram (ECG) signals. ECG is a non-invasive method for measuring the electrical activity of the heart over time. It provides valuable information about the heart's rhythm, rate, and any abnormalities. MATLAB provides powerful tools for processing and analyzing ECG signals.

Objective

The objective of this case study is to demonstrate the use of MATLAB for ECG signal analysis. We will load an ECG signal, preprocess it, extract relevant features, and perform basic analysis tasks.

Step 1: Loading the ECG Signal

First, we need to load the ECG signal into MATLAB. Assume we have an ECG signal stored in a .mat file named "ecg_data.mat". We can load the signal using the load function:

```
load('ecg_data.mat');
```

Step 2: Preprocessing the ECG Signal

Before analyzing the ECG signal, we may need to preprocess it to remove noise and baseline wander. MATLAB provides functions for signal filtering and detrending.

```
fs = 360; % Sampling frequency in Hz
fc = 50; % Cutoff frequency for high-pass filter
[b, a] = butter(4, fc/(fs/2), 'high'); % Design a high-pass Butterworth filter
filtered_ecg = filtfilt(b, a, ecg_data); % Apply the filter to remove baseline wander

detrended_ecg = detrend(filtered_ecg); % Remove any linear trend
```

Step 3: Extracting ECG Features

Next, we can extract relevant features from the ECG signal, such as R-peak locations, heart rate, and QRS duration. MATLAB provides the findpeaks function for detecting peaks in the signal.

```
[peaks, locations] = findpeaks(detrended_ecg, 'MinPeakHeight', 0.5, 'MinPeakDistance', 0.3*fs);
rr_intervals = diff(locations) / fs; % Calculate R-R intervals in seconds
heart_rate = 60 ./ rr_intervals; % Calculate heart rate in beats per minute
```

Step 4: Plotting the ECG Signal and Features

We can visualize the ECG signal and the extracted features using MATLAB's plotting functions.

```
time = (0:length(ecg_data)-1) / fs; % Create a time vector
figure;
subplot(2, 1, 1);
plot(time, ecg_data);
title('Raw ECG Signal');
xlabel('Time (s)');
ylabel('Amplitude');

subplot(2, 1, 2);
plot(time, detrended_ecg);
hold on;
plot(locations/fs, peaks, 'ro', 'MarkerFaceColor', 'r');
title('Detrended ECG Signal with R-Peaks');
xlabel('Time (s)');
ylabel('Amplitude');
```

Step 5: Analyzing ECG Features

Finally, we can perform basic analysis tasks on the extracted features, such as calculating average heart rate, detecting abnormalities, or classifying ECG beats.

```
average_heart_rate = mean(heart_rate);
fprintf('Average Heart Rate: %.2f beats per minute\n', average_heart_rate);

% Perform further analysis tasks based on specific requirements
```

This case study demonstrates a simple workflow for ECG signal analysis using MATLAB. It covers loading the signal, preprocessing it, extracting features, visualizing the results, and performing basic analysis tasks.

MATLAB provides a wide range of functions and toolboxes for more advanced ECG signal analysis, including:

Wavelet-based denoising

QRS complex detection and segmentation

Heart rate variability analysis

rrhythmia detection and classification

Case Study 2: Brain Tumor Segmentation from MRI Images

Objective

The objective of this case study is to demonstrate the use of MATLAB for segmenting brain tumors from magnetic resonance imaging (MRI) scans. We will load an MRI image, preprocess it, apply image segmentation techniques, and visualize the segmented tumor region.

Step 1: Loading the MRI Image

First, we load the MRI image into MATLAB using the imread function.

```
mri_image = imread('brain_mri.jpg');
```

Step 2: Preprocessing the MRI Image

Before segmenting the tumor, we preprocess the MRI image to enhance its quality and remove noise.

```
gray_image = rgb2gray(mri_image); % Convert the image to grayscale
filtered_image = medfilt2(gray_image, [5, 5]); % Apply median filtering
enhanced_image = imadjust(filtered_image); % Adjust the contrast
```

Step 3: Tumor Segmentation

We apply image segmentation techniques to isolate the tumor region from the enhanced MRI image.

```
threshold = graythresh(enhanced_image); % Compute the optimal threshold using Otsu's method
```

binary_image = imbinarize(enhanced_image, threshold); % Convert the image to binary
labeled_image = bwlabel(binary_image); % Label connected components
tumor_region = labeled_image == 1; % Assume the largest connected component is the tumor

Step 4: Visualizing the Segmented Tumor

We can visualize the segmented tumor region by overlaying it on the original MRI image.

segmented_image = imoverlay(mri_image, tumor_region, [1, 0, 0]); % Overlay the tumor region in red
imshow(segmented_image);
title('Segmented Brain Tumor');

This case study demonstrates a basic workflow for brain tumor segmentation using MATLAB. It covers loading the MRI image, preprocessing it, applying segmentation techniques, and visualizing the segmented tumor region.

MATLAB provides additional functions and toolboxes for more advanced tumor segmentation tasks, such as:

Fuzzy C-means clustering
Region growing algorithms
Deep learning-based segmentation using convolutional neural networks

Case Study 3: Respiratory Rate Estimation from Photoplethysmogram (PPG) Signals

Objective:

The objective of this case study is to demonstrate the use of MATLAB for estimating the respiratory rate from photoplethysmogram (PPG) signals. PPG is a non-invasive optical technique that measures changes in blood volume in the tissue. The respiratory activity modulates the PPG signal, allowing for the estimation of the respiratory rate.

Step 1: Loading the PPG Signal

We load the PPG signal into MATLAB from a .mat file.

load('ppg_signal.mat');

Step 2: Preprocessing the PPG Signal

We preprocess the PPG signal to remove noise and baseline wander.

```
fs = 100; % Sampling frequency in Hz
fc = 0.5; % Cutoff frequency for high-pass filter
[b, a] = butter(4, fc/(fs/2), 'high'); % Design a high-pass Butterworth filter
filtered_ppg = filtfilt(b, a, ppg_signal); % Apply the filter to remove baseline wander
```

Step 3: Estimating the Respiratory Rate

We estimate the respiratory rate from the filtered PPG signal using the power spectral density (PSD) analysis.

```
window_size = 30 * fs; % 30-second window size
overlap = 15 * fs; % 15-second overlap
[psd, f] = pwelch(filtered_ppg, window_size, overlap, [], fs); % Compute the PSD
respiratory_band = (f >= 0.1) & (f <= 0.4); % Respiratory frequency band (0.1-0.4 Hz)
[~, max_idx] = max(psd(respiratory_band)); % Find the peak frequency in the respiratory band
respiratory_rate = f(find(respiratory_band, 1) + max_idx - 1) * 60; % Convert to breaths per minute
```

Step 4: Visualizing the Results

We can plot the PPG signal and the estimated respiratory rate.

```
time = (0:length(ppg_signal)-1) / fs; % Create a time vector
figure;
subplot(2, 1, 1);
plot(time, ppg_signal);
title('Raw PPG Signal');
xlabel('Time (s)');
ylabel('Amplitude');

subplot(2, 1, 2);
plot(time, filtered_ppg);
title(sprintf('Filtered PPG Signal (Estimated Respiratory Rate: %.2f breaths/min)', respiratory_rate));
xlabel('Time (s)');
```

ylabel('Amplitude');

This case study demonstrates a simple approach to estimate the respiratory rate from PPG signals using MATLAB. It covers loading the PPG signal, preprocessing it, estimating the respiratory rate using PSD analysis, and visualizing the results.

MATLAB offers additional techniques and algorithms for respiratory rate estimation, such as:

Time-domain analysis (e.g., peak detection, zero-crossing)

Wavelet transform-based methods

Empirical mode decomposition (EMD)

Deep learning-based approaches

15 RUST PROGRAMMING FOR SECURE AND EFFICIENT HEALTHCARE SYSTEMS

15.1 Introduction to Rust Programming

Rust is a systems programming language that focuses on safety, concurrency, and memory efficiency. It has gained significant popularity in recent years due to its ability to prevent common programming errors, such as null or dangling pointer dereferences, buffer overflows, and data races. Rust's unique ownership system and borrow checker ensure memory safety at compile-time, eliminating entire classes of bugs that can lead to security vulnerabilities and crashes.

In the context of healthcare systems, where security, reliability, and performance are critical, Rust provides a compelling choice for developing robust and efficient applications. Its strong static typing, extensive compile-time checks, and built-in support for concurrency make it well-suited for building secure and scalable healthcare software.

15.2 Key Features of Rust:
15.2.1 Memory Safety
a. Rust's ownership system and borrow checker enforce strict rules for memory management at compile-time.

b. It prevents common memory-related bugs, such as null or dangling pointer dereferences and buffer overflows.

c. Rust's memory safety guarantees reduce the risk of security vulnerabilities and crashes.

15.2.2. Concurrency
a. Rust provides built-in support for concurrent programming through its ownership system and safe concurrency primitives.

b. It allows developers to write concurrent code without the risk of data races or other synchronization issues.

c. Rust's concurrency model enables efficient utilization of system resources and supports scalable healthcare applications.

15.2.3. Performance
a. Rust is designed to be a systems programming language with minimal runtime overhead.

b. It offers fine-grained control over system resources and memory layout.

c. Rust's zero-cost abstractions and ability to leverage

low-level optimizations enable the development of high-performance healthcare systems.

15.2.4. Interoperability

a. Rust provides seamless interoperability with C and other languages through its foreign function interface (FFI).

b. It allows integration with existing healthcare systems, libraries, and frameworks written in other languages.

c. Rust can be used to write performance-critical components that interface with existing healthcare infrastructure.

15.2.5. Strong Static Typing:

a. Rust has a strong static type system that catches many errors at compile-time.

b. It enforces type safety and reduces the chances of runtime errors and unexpected behavior.

c. Rust's type system helps in writing more reliable and maintainable healthcare software.

15.3 Getting Started with Rust:

To start developing with Rust, you need to install the Rust toolchain on your system. The official Rust website (https://www.rust-lang.org/) provides installation instructions for different operating systems.

Once installed, you can use the Rust package manager, Cargo, to create a new Rust project:

```
cargo new healthcare_project
cd healthcare_project
```

Rust source files have the .rs extension, and the entry point of a Rust program is the main function in the main.rs file:

```
fn main() {
    println!("Hello, Rust for Healthcare!");
}
```

You can build and run the project using Cargo:
cargo run

Rust has a growing ecosystem of libraries and frameworks that can be leveraged for healthcare application development. The Rust package registry, crates.io, hosts a wide range of packages covering various domains, including networking, databases, cryptography, and data processing.

Learning Rust programming and applying its principles to healthcare systems development can help create secure, efficient, and reliable applications. Rust's memory safety guarantees, concurrency support, and performance optimizations make it a valuable tool in the healthcare software development toolkit.

In the following sections, we will explore more specific topics related to developing high-performance and memory-safe healthcare applications using Rust.

15.4 Developing High-Performance and Memory-Safe Applications

Rust's unique features and design principles make it well-suited for developing high-performance and memory-safe healthcare applications. Let's explore some key aspects of Rust that contribute to building efficient and secure software.

15.4.1. Ownership and Borrowing

Rust's ownership system ensures that there is exactly one owner for each piece of data at any given time. The owner is responsible for freeing the memory associated with the data when it goes out of scope. Rust's borrow checker enforces strict rules for borrowing references to data, preventing data races and other memory-related issues.

Rust eliminates common memory safety bugs and ensures efficient memory management by adhering to these rules.

Example:

```
fn main() {
    let data = vec![1, 2, 3, 4, 5];
```

```
    let borrowed_data = &data;
    println!("Borrowed data: {:?}", borrowed_data);
    // The borrowed reference goes out of scope here
}
// The owner `data` is automatically deallocated here
```

15.4.2 Concurrency and Parallelism

Rust provides safe and efficient concurrency primitives, such as threads, mutexes, and channels.

The ownership system and borrow checker extend to concurrent code, preventing data races and ensuring thread safety.

Rust's std::sync module offers synchronization primitives like Mutex and RwLock for safe shared mutable state.

The std::thread module allows creating and managing threads for concurrent execution.

Rust's concurrency model enables developers to write parallel and asynchronous code without sacrificing safety.

Example:

```
use std::sync::{Arc, Mutex};
use std::thread;

fn main() {
    let shared_data = Arc::new(Mutex::new(0));
    let mut handles = vec![];

    for _ in 0..5 {
        let data = Arc::clone(&shared_data);
        let handle = thread::spawn(move || {
            let mut value = data.lock().unwrap();
            *value += 1;
        });
        handles.push(handle);
    }

    for handle in handles {
        handle.join().unwrap();
    }

    println!("Result: {}", *shared_data.lock().unwrap());
```

```
}
```

15.4.3 Performance Optimization

Rust's zero-cost abstractions allow developers to write high-level, expressive code without sacrificing performance. Rust's static dispatch and monomorphization enable efficient code generation and optimization. The Rust compiler performs extensive optimizations, such as inlining, dead code elimination, and loop unrolling. Rust's fine-grained control over memory layout and allocation enables low-level optimizations when needed. Profiling and benchmarking tools, such as cargo-bench and perf, can be used to measure and optimize the performance of Rust code.

Example:

```
fn process_data(data: &[u32]) -> u32 {
    data.iter().fold(0, |acc, &x| acc + x)
}

fn main() {
    let data = vec![1, 2, 3, 4, 5];
    let result = process_data(&data);
    println!("Result: {}", result);
}
```

15.4.4. Error Handling and Type Safety

Rust's type system and error handling mechanisms promote writing robust and reliable code. The Result and Option types are used for explicit error handling and expressing the possibility of absence. Rust's match expressions provide exhaustive pattern matching, ensuring all possible cases are handled. The #[must_use] attribute can be used to enforce the handling of important return values.

Rust's strong typing and compile-time checks catch many errors before runtime, reducing the chances of unexpected behavior.

Example:

```
fn divide(a: i32, b: i32) -> Result<i32, String> {
    if b == 0 {
        Err(String::from("Division by zero"))
    } else {
```

```
        Ok(a / b)
      }
   }
   fn main() {
      match divide(10, 2) {
         Ok(result) => println!("Result: {}", result),
         Err(err) => println!("Error: {}", err),
      }

      match divide(10, 0) {
         Ok(result) => println!("Result: {}", result),
         Err(err) => println!("Error: {}", err),
      }
   }
```

These are just a few examples of how Rust's features and principles can be applied to develop high-performance and memory-safe healthcare applications. Rust's ownership system, concurrency support, and performance optimizations enable developers to write efficient and secure code.

When building healthcare systems with Rust, it's essential to leverage Rust's ecosystem and best practices. Utilizing well-established libraries and frameworks, such as tokio for asynchronous programming, serde for serialization and deserialization, and diesel for database access, can greatly enhance productivity and code quality.

Additionally, following Rust's coding guidelines, writing comprehensive tests, and conducting thorough code reviews can help ensure the reliability and maintainability of healthcare applications.

Case Study 1: Building a Secure Telemedicine Platform

Objective

In this case study, we will explore how Rust can be used to build a secure and efficient telemedicine platform. The platform will enable patients to consult with doctors remotely, ensuring the privacy and security of sensitive medical data.

Step 1: System Architecture

We'll design a system architecture that consists of the following components:

a. Patient Application: A web-based application for patients to schedule appointments and interact with doctors.

b. Doctor Application: A web-based application for doctors to manage appointments and communicate with patients.

c. Backend Server: A Rust-based server that handles data storage, authentication, and communication between the patient and doctor applications.

d. Database: A secure database for storing patient records, appointment details, and other relevant information.

Step 2: Implementing the Backend Server

We'll use Rust to implement the backend server, utilizing its memory safety and concurrency features.

```rust
use actix_web::{web, App, HttpServer};
use sqlx::PgPool;

async fn main() -> std::io::Result<()> {
    let database_url = "postgres://username:password@localhost/telemedicine";
    let pool = PgPool::new(&database_url).await.unwrap();

    HttpServer::new(move || {
        App::new()
            .data(pool.clone())
            .route("/api/appointments", web::get().to(get_appointments))
            .route("/api/appointments", web::post().to(create_appointment))
            // Add more routes for authentication, patient management, etc.
    })
    .bind("127.0.0.1:8080")?
    .run()
    .await
}
```

Step 3: Implementing Authentication and Authorization

We'll use Rust's jsonwebtoken crate to implement secure

authentication and authorization.

```rust
use jsonwebtoken::{encode, decode, Header, Algorithm, Validation};

fn create_token(user_id: i32) -> String {
    let claims = Claims {
        sub: user_id.to_string(),
        exp: (Utc::now() + Duration::hours(1)).timestamp() as usize,
    };
    encode(&Header::default(), &claims, &EncodingKey::from_secret("secret".as_ref())).unwrap()
}

fn validate_token(token: &str) -> Result<i32, jsonwebtoken::errors::Error> {
    let validation = Validation::default();
    let token_data = decode::<Claims>(token, &DecodingKey::from_secret("secret".as_ref()), &validation)?;
    Ok(token_data.claims.sub.parse().unwrap())
}
```

Step 4: Implementing Secure Communication

We'll use the rustls crate to enable secure communication between the patient and doctor applications and the backend server.

```rust
use rustls::ServerConfig;
use actix_web::HttpServer;
use actix_rustls::RustlsServer;

async fn main() -> std::io::Result<()> {
    let config = ServerConfig::new(NoClientAuth::new());
    HttpServer::new(|| {
        App::new()
            // Application routes and middleware
    })
    .bind_rustls("127.0.0.1:8443", config)?
    .run()
    .await
}
```

Step 5: Implementing Data Encryption

We'll use the ring crate to encrypt sensitive patient data before storing it in the database.

```
use ring::{aead, rand};

fn encrypt_data(data: &[u8], key: &[u8]) -> Vec<u8> {
    let nonce = rand::generate(&mut rand::SystemRandom::new()).unwrap();
    let mut buffer = data.to_vec();
    buffer.extend_from_slice(&nonce);
    let sealing_key = aead::SealingKey::new(&aead::CHACHA20_POLY1305, key).unwrap();
    let sealed_data = aead::seal_in_place(&sealing_key, &nonce, &[], &mut buffer, 16).unwrap();
    sealed_data.to_vec()
}
```

We can build a secure telemedicine platform that ensures the confidentiality and integrity of patient data by utilizing Rust's security features and libraries. Rust's memory safety guarantees and strong typing help prevent common security vulnerabilities, while its concurrency primitives enable efficient handling of multiple client connections.

The use of secure authentication, encrypted communication, and data encryption techniques further enhances the overall security of the telemedicine system.

Case Study 2: Developing a High-Performance Medical Image Processing Pipeline

Objective

In this case study, we will explore how Rust can be used to develop a high-performance medical image processing pipeline. The pipeline will efficiently process and analyze large volumes of medical images, such as MRI scans or X-rays, to assist in diagnosis and treatment planning.

Step 1: Designing the Image Processing Pipeline

We'll design a modular and extensible image processing pipeline that consists of the following stages:

a. Image Loading: Loading medical images from various file formats (e.g., DICOM, NIFTI).

b.Preprocessing: Applying image preprocessing techniques, such as noise reduction and intensity normalization.

c. Segmentation: Segmenting regions of interest (ROIs)

from the medical images.

d. Feature Extraction: Extracting relevant features from the segmented ROIs.

e. Classification: Classifying the extracted features to assist in diagnosis or treatment planning.

Step 2: Implementing Image Loading

We'll use the dcm-rs crate to load DICOM images and the nifti crate to load NIFTI images.

```rust
use dcm::DcmFileIO;
use nifti::NiftiObject;
fn load_dicom_image(file_path: &str) -> Result<Vec<u16>,
dcm::DcmError> {
    let mut file = DcmFileIO::open(file_path)?;
    let dataset = file.read_dataset()?;
    let pixel_data = dataset.elements().find(|e| e.tag() ==
dcm::tags::PIXEL_DATA).unwrap();
    let pixel_data = pixel_data.value().as_bytes().unwrap();
    Ok(pixel_data.chunks(2).map(|c| u16::from_le_bytes([c[0],
c[1]])).collect())
}

fn load_nifti_image(file_path: &str) -> Result<NiftiObject,
nifti::Error> {
    let nifti_object = NiftiObject::from_file(file_path)?;
    Ok(nifti_object)
}
```

Step 3: Implementing Image Preprocessing

We'll use the image crate for basic image processing tasks and the ndarray crate for efficient multi-dimensional array operations.

```rust
use image::{GrayImage, imageops};
use ndarray::{Array3, Axis};
fn preprocess_image(image: &GrayImage) -> Array3<f32> {
    let normalized_image = imageops::normalize(image);
    let array = Array3::from_shape_vec(
        (normalized_image.height()                as           usize,
normalized_image.width() as usize, 1),
        normalized_image.to_vec(),
    ).unwrap();
    array.map(|&x| x as f32 / 255.0)
}
```

Step 4: Implementing Image Segmentation

We'll use the imageproc crate for image segmentation algorithms, such as thresholding and region growing.

```
use imageproc::morphology::dilate;
use imageproc::region_labelling::connected_components;
fn segment_image(image: &Array3<f32>, threshold: f32) ->
Array3<u32> {
    let binary_image = image.map(|&x| if x > threshold { 255 }
else { 0 });
    let dilated_image = dilate(&binary_image.map(|&x| x as u8),
3);
    let labeled_image = connected_components(&dilated_image);
    labeled_image.map(|&x| x as u32)
}
```

Step 5: Implementing Feature Extraction and Classification

We'll use the rustlearn crate for machine learning algorithms, such as feature extraction and classification.

```
use rustlearn::prelude::*;
use rustlearn::feature_extraction::PCA;
use rustlearn::svm::SVC;
fn extract_features(segmented_image: &Array3<u32>) ->
Array2<f64> {
    let                     flattened_image                  =
segmented_image.view().into_iter().map(|&x|        x        as
f64).collect::<Vec<_>>();
    let pca = PCA::default().set_n_components(50);
    let features = pca.fit_transform(&Array2::from_shape_vec((1,
flattened_image.len()), flattened_image).unwrap()).unwrap();
    features
}

fn classify_features(features: &Array2<f64>, model: &SVC) ->
usize {
    model.predict(features).unwrap()
}
```

We can develop a medical image processing pipeline that can handle large volumes of data with optimal resource utilization by utilizing Rust's high-performance libraries and efficient memory management. Rust's concurrency primitives, such as threads and rayon, enable parallel processing of images, further enhancing the pipeline's performance.

The modular design of the pipeline allows for easy extension and customization, accommodating different image formats, preprocessing techniques, segmentation algorithms, and classification models.

Rust's strong type system and compile-time checks ensure the correctness and reliability of the image processing code, reducing the chances of runtime errors and unexpected behavior.

Case Study 3: Implementing a Secure and Efficient Electronic Health Record (EHR) System

Objective

In this case study, we will explore how Rust can be used to implement a secure and efficient Electronic Health Record (EHR) system. The EHR system will store and manage patient medical records, ensuring the confidentiality, integrity, and availability of sensitive healthcare data.

Step 1: Designing the EHR System Architecture

We'll design a scalable and modular EHR system architecture that consists of the following components:

a. EHR Server: A Rust-based server that handles data storage, retrieval, and access control.

b. EHR Database: A secure database for storing patient medical records and related information.

c. EHR API: A well-defined API for interacting with the EHR system, supporting CRUD operations on medical records.

d. Authentication and Authorization: Mechanisms for secure user authentication and role-based access control.

Step 2: Implementing the EHR Server

We'll use the actix-web framework to build the EHR server and the diesel ORM for database integration.

```
use actix_web::{web, App, HttpServer};
use diesel::{PgConnection, r2d2::{self, ConnectionManager}};

type             DbPool             =
r2d2::Pool<ConnectionManager<PgConnection>>;
```

```rust
async fn main() -> std::io::Result<()> {
    let database_url = "postgres://username:password@localhost/ehr";
    let manager = ConnectionManager::<PgConnection>::new(database_url);
    let pool = r2d2::Pool::builder().build(manager).unwrap();

    HttpServer::new(move || {
        App::new()
          .data(pool.clone())
          .route("/api/patients", web::get().to(get_patients))
          .route("/api/patients", web::post().to(create_patient))
          // Add more routes for medical record management
    })
    .bind("127.0.0.1:8080")?
    .run()
    .await
}
```

Step 3: Implementing Authentication and Authorization

We'll use the jsonwebtoken crate for JWT-based authentication and the casbin crate for role-based access control (RBAC).

```rust
use jsonwebtoken::{encode, decode, Header, Algorithm, Validation};
use casbin::{Enforcer, DefaultModel, FileAdapter};

fn create_token(user_id: i32, role: &str) -> String {
    let claims = Claims {
        sub: user_id.to_string(),
        role: role.to_string(),
        exp: (Utc::now() + Duration::hours(1)).timestamp() as usize,
    };
    encode(&Header::default(), &claims, &EncodingKey::from_secret("secret".as_ref())).unwrap()
}

fn authorize(enforcer: &Enforcer, role: &str, resource: &str, action: &str) -> bool {
    enforcer.enforce((role, resource, action)).unwrap()
}
```

Step 4: Implementing Secure Data Storage

We'll use the ring crate for data encryption and the sha2

crate for hashing sensitive information.

```rust
use ring::{aead, rand};
use sha2::{Sha256, Digest};

fn encrypt_data(data: &[u8], key: &[u8]) -> Vec<u8> {
    // Same encryption code as in the telemedicine case study
}

fn hash_password(password: &str) -> String {
    let mut hasher = Sha256::new();
    hasher.update(password.as_bytes());
    format!("{:x}", hasher.finalize())
}
```

Step 5: Implementing the EHR API

We'll define a RESTful API for interacting with the EHR system, supporting CRUD operations on patient medical records.

```rust
use actix_web::{web, HttpResponse};
use serde::{Deserialize, Serialize};

#[derive(Deserialize)]
struct CreatePatient {
    name: String,
    age: i32,
    // Other patient fields
}

#[derive(Serialize)]
struct Patient {
    id: i32,
    name: String,
    age: i32,
    // Other patient fields
}

async fn get_patients(pool: web::Data<DbPool>) -> HttpResponse {
    // Retrieve patients from the database
    // Serialize and return the patients
}

async fn create_patient(pool: web::Data<DbPool>, patient: web::Json<CreatePatient>) -> HttpResponse {
    // Insert the new patient into the database
```

```
    // Return the created patient
}
```

We can build an EHR system that ensures the protection of sensitive patient data by utilizing Rust's security features, such as secure encryption and hashing, along with robust authentication and authorization mechanisms. Rust's memory safety guarantees and strong typing help prevent common vulnerabilities and ensure the integrity of the EHR application.

The use of Rust's efficient concurrency primitives and asynchronous programming model allows for high-performance handling of multiple client requests and optimal resource utilization.

The modular architecture of the EHR system enables easy integration with existing healthcare systems and facilitates future scalability and extensibility.

Rust's powerful ecosystem, including web frameworks, database libraries, and security-related crates, provides a solid foundation for building secure and efficient healthcare applications.

16 JULIA PROGRAMMING FOR SCIENTIFIC COMPUTING IN HEALTHCARE

16.1 Introduction to Julia Programming

Julia is a high-level, high-performance programming language designed for scientific computing and numerical analysis. It combines the ease of use and expressiveness of Python with the performance of low-level languages like C and Fortran. Julia's unique features make it well-suited for scientific computing tasks in healthcare, such as data analysis, machine learning, and computational modeling.

16.2 Key Features of Julia

High Performance: Julia is designed for speed and efficiency. It utilizes a just-in-time (JIT) compiler, which allows it to achieve performance comparable to low-level languages while maintaining the simplicity and ease of use of high-level languages.

Dynamic Typing: Julia supports dynamic typing, which means that variable types are determined at runtime. This allows for flexibility and rapid prototyping, making it easier to write and modify code.

Multiple Dispatch: Julia employs a powerful feature called multiple dispatch, which enables efficient and expressive code. It allows functions to be defined with different behavior based on the types of their arguments, leading to cleaner and more readable code.

Metaprogramming: Julia provides metaprogramming capabilities, allowing developers to write code that generates or manipulates other code. This enables the creation of domain-specific languages (DSLs) and powerful abstractions

Extensive ecosystem: Julia has a growing ecosystem of libraries and packages specifically tailored for scientific computing, including packages for linear algebra, optimization, statistics, machine learning, and visualization

16.2 Getting Started with Julia

16.2.1 Installation: Julia can be downloaded and installed from the official Julia website (https://julialang.org). It is available for Windows, macOS, and Linux.

16.2.2 REPL: Once installed, you can start the Julia REPL (Read-Eval-Print Loop) by typing julia in the terminal. The REPL provides an interactive environment for executing Julia code.

16.2.3 Packages: Julia has a built-in package manager that allows you to easily install and manage packages. You can access the package manager by typing] in the REPL, which switches to the package mode. To install a package, simply type add PackageName.

16.2.4 IDE Support: While the REPL is suitable for quick experimentation, you can also use integrated development environments (IDEs) for more advanced development. Popular IDEs with Julia support include Juno, VS Code with the Julia extension, and JupyterLab.

16.3 Basic Syntax and Data Types

16.3.1 Variables: In Julia, variables are declared using the = operator. For example: x = 10.

16.3.2 Data Types: Julia supports various data types, including integers (Int), floating-point numbers (Float64), booleans (Bool), strings (String), and arrays (Array).

16.3.3 Functions: Functions in Julia are defined using the function keyword, followed by the function name, arguments, and the function body.

For example:

```
function add(a, b)
    return a + b
end
```

16.3.4 Control Flow: Julia provides standard control flow constructs like if-else statements, for loops, and while loops.

16.3.5 Arrays: Arrays in Julia are 1-based, meaning the first element is accessed with an index of 1. You can create an array using square brackets: arr = [1, 2, 3].

Example: Basic Data Analysis in Julia. Let's consider a simple example of performing basic data analysis on a dataset of patient ages:

```
# Create an array of patient ages
ages = [25, 30, 45, 28, 52, 36, 41, 29, 33, 47]
# Calculate the mean age
mean_age = sum(ages) / length(ages)
println("Mean age: ", mean_age)
# Calculate the median age
sorted_ages = sort(ages)
median_age   =   length(ages)   %   2   ==   0   ?
(sorted_ages[length(ages)÷2] + sorted_ages[length(ages)÷2+1])
/ 2 : sorted_ages[length(ages)÷2+1]
println("Median age: ", median_age)
# Calculate the age range
age_range = maximum(ages) - minimum(ages)
println("Age range: ", age_range)
Output:
Mean age: 36.6
Median age: 34.0
Age range: 27
```

In this example, we create an array of patient ages and perform basic statistical calculations such as mean, median, and range using built-in Julia functions. Julia's simplicity, performance, and growing ecosystem make it an attractive choice for scientific computing tasks in healthcare. Its ability to handle large datasets, complex computations, and numerical simulations efficiently can greatly benefit healthcare researchers and data scientists. Learning Julia and applying it to healthcare-related projects can open up new possibilities for data analysis, predictive modeling, and computational simulations

16.4 Numerical Computing and Optimization

Numerical computing and optimization are fundamental aspects of scientific computing in healthcare. Julia provides powerful tools and libraries for performing numerical computations and solving optimization problems efficiently.

16.4.1 Linear Algebra: Julia has built-in support for linear algebra operations through the LinearAlgebra standard library. It provides functions for matrix and vector operations, eigenvalue problems, factorizations, and more. Example:

```julia
using LinearAlgebra
A = [1 2; 3 4]
b = [5, 6]
x = A \ b  # Solve the linear system Ax = b
```

Optimization: Julia offers several optimization libraries, such as Optim and JuMP, for solving optimization problems. These libraries provide algorithms for unconstrained and constrained optimization, linear programming, nonlinear programming, and more. Example using Optim:

```julia
using Optim
function objective(x)
    return (x[1] - 1)^2 + (x[2] - 2)^2
end
initial_guess = [0.0, 0.0]
result = optimize(objective, initial_guess, BFGS())
```

Differential Equations: Julia has a robust ecosystem for solving differential equations, which is essential in many healthcare applications.

The DifferentialEquations package provides a wide range of solvers for ordinary differential equations (ODEs), stochastic differential equations (SDEs), delay differential equations (DDEs), and more. Example:

using DifferentialEquations

```julia
function lorenz(du, u, p, t)
    du[1] = 10.0 * (u[2] - u[1])
    du[2] = u[1] * (28.0 - u[3]) - u[2]
    du[3] = u[1] * u[2] - (8/3) * u[3]
end
u0 = [1.0, 0.0, 0.0]
tspan = (0.0, 100.0)
prob = ODEProblem(lorenz, u0, tspan)
sol = solve(prob)
```

Parallel Computing: Julia supports parallel computing, allowing you to leverage multi-core processors and distributed computing environments. The Distributed standard library provides functionality for distributed computing, while the Threads module enables multi-threading. Example:

```
using Distributed
addprocs(4)  # Add 4 worker processes
@distributed for i in 1:10
   # Perform parallel computation
   result = expensive_computation(i)
   # Collect results
end
```

16.5 Case Study 1: Modeling Pharmacokinetics and Pharmacodynamics

Pharmacokinetics (PK) and pharmacodynamics (PD) are essential concepts in drug development and clinical pharmacology. PK describes how the body processes a drug, while PD describes the drug's effect on the body. Modeling PK and PD helps in understanding drug behavior, optimizing dosing regimens, and predicting drug responses.

Let's consider a simple example of modeling the concentration of a drug in the body over time using a one-compartment model with first-order absorption and elimination. We'll use Julia and the Differential Equations package to solve the ordinary differential equation (ODE) representing the model.

```
using DifferentialEquations
using Plots
# Model parameters
ka = 0.5  # Absorption rate constant
```

```
ke = 0.2  # Elimination rate constant
Dose = 100  # Drug dose
# ODE function
function one_compartment_model(du, u, p, t)
    ka, ke, Dose = p
    du[1] = -ka * u[1]
    du[2] = ka * u[1] - ke * u[2]
end
# Initial conditions
u0 = [Dose, 0.0]
# Time span
tspan = (0.0, 24.0)
# Parameter vector
p = [ka, ke, Dose]
# Define the ODE problem
prob = ODEProblem(one_compartment_model, u0, tspan, p)
# Solve the ODE
sol = solve(prob)
# Plot the solution
plot(sol, label=["Gut"  "Plasma"], xlabel="Time (hours)",
ylabel="Concentration")
```

In this example, we define the one-compartment model using an ODE function. The model parameters include the absorption rate constant (ka), elimination rate constant (ke), and the drug dose (Dose). The ODE function describes the change in drug concentration in the gut and plasma compartments over time.

We set the initial conditions (u0) to represent the drug dose in the gut compartment and zero concentration in the plasma compartment. We also specify the time span (tspan) over which we want to simulate the model. Using the ODE Problem function from the Differential Equations package, we define the ODE problem by passing the ODE function, initial conditions, time span, and parameter vector. We then solve the ODE using the solve function. Finally, we plot the solution to visualize the drug concentration in the gut and plasma compartments over time. This case study demonstrates how Julia can be used to model and simulate pharmacokinetic and pharmacodynamic processes.

Researchers and practitioners can develop more complex PK/PD models, perform parameter estimation, and optimize drug dosing regimens by utilizing Julia's numerical computing capabilities and the extensive ecosystem of libraries.

Julia's high performance and ease of use make it a valuable tool for modeling and simulation in drug development and clinical pharmacology. Its ability to handle large-scale simulations and its seamless integration with optimization techniques enable researchers to explore and analyze various scenarios efficiently

Case Study 2: Image Segmentation for Medical Image Analysis

Medical image analysis often involves segmenting images to identify and extract specific regions of interest, such as tumors or organs. Julia's image processing capabilities and machine learning libraries make it well-suited for this task.

Let's consider an example of segmenting a brain MRI image to extract the tumor region using the Images and Clustering packages in Julia.

```
using Images
using Clustering
# Load the brain MRI image
image = load("brain_mri.jpg")
# Convert the image to grayscale
gray_image = Gray.(image)
# Reshape the image into a vector of pixel intensities
data = reshape(float.(gray_image), :, size(gray_image, 3))
# Perform k-means clustering with 3 clusters
k = 3
result = kmeans(data, k)
# Create a segmented image based on cluster assignments
```

```
segmented_image                =                map(i                ->
RGB(result.centers[result.assignments[i],                        :]),
1:length(result.assignments))
segmented_image        =                reshape(segmented_image,
size(gray_image))
# Display the original and segmented images
plot(gray_image, title="Original Image")
plot(segmented_image, title="Segmented Image")
```

In this example, we load a brain MRI image and convert it to grayscale using the Images package. We then reshape the image into a vector of pixel intensities.

Next, we perform k-means clustering on the pixel intensities using the Clustering package. We specify the number of clusters (k) as 3, assuming that the image consists of three main regions: background, healthy tissue, and tumor.

After clustering, we create a segmented image by assigning each pixel to its corresponding cluster center. We use different colors to represent each cluster in the segmented image.

Finally, we display the original grayscale image and the segmented image side by side using the plot function. This case study demonstrates how Julia can be used for medical image segmentation tasks. Researchers can develop automated segmentation pipelines to extract regions of interest from medical images by utilizing image processing libraries and clustering algorithms. Julia's performance and flexibility make it suitable for handling large datasets and complex image analysis tasks.

Case Study 3: Predicting Patient Readmission using Machine Learning

Predicting patient readmission is an important task in healthcare analytics. It involves identifying patients who are at high risk of being readmitted to the hospital within a certain timeframe after discharge. Julia's machine learning capabilities can be utilized to build predictive models for patient readmission.

Let's consider an example of building a logistic regression model to predict patient readmission using the GLM package in Julia.

```julia
using GLM
using DataFrames
using CSV
# Load the patient readmission dataset
data = CSV.read("patient_readmission.csv", DataFrame)
# Preprocess the data
data[!, :Age] = 2023 .- data[!, :YearOfBirth]
data[!, :Readmitted] = ifelse.(data[!, :DaysToReadmission] .<= 30, 1, 0)
select!(data, Not(:DaysToReadmission))
# Split the data into features and target variable
features = select(data, Not(:Readmitted))
target = data[!, :Readmitted]
# Fit a logistic regression model
model = glm(@formula(Readmitted ~ Age + NumDiagnoses + NumProcedures + NumLabs), data, Binomial(), LogitLink())
# Make predictions on new data
new_data = DataFrame(Age=[65, 50], NumDiagnoses=[3, 2], NumProcedures=[2, 1], NumLabs=[10, 8])
predictions = predict(model, new_data)
# Print the predicted probabilities
println(predictions)
```

In this example, we load a patient readmission dataset from a CSV file into a DataFrame using the CSV and DataFrames packages.

We preprocess the data by calculating the age from the year of birth and creating a binary target variable indicating whether the patient was readmitted within 30 days or not. We also select relevant features for the predictive model.

Next, we fit a logistic regression model using the glm function from the GLM package. We specify the formula that relates the target variable (Readmitted) to the selected features

(Age, NumDiagnoses, NumProcedures, NumLabs).

After training the model, we can make predictions on new data. We create a DataFrame with new patient information and use the predict function to obtain the predicted probabilities of readmission.

Finally, we print the predicted probabilities for the new patients. This case study showcases how Julia can be used for predictive modeling tasks in healthcare. Researchers can build models to predict patient outcomes, such as readmission risk by utilizing machine learning libraries like GLM. Julia's performance and ease of use make it suitable for handling large datasets and complex modeling tasks.

17 SWIFT PROGRAMMING FOR MOBILE HEALTHCARE APP DEVELOPMENT

Swift is a modern, powerful, and intuitive programming language developed by Apple for building apps across their ecosystem, including iOS, iPadOS, macOS, watchOS, and tvOS. Swift is designed to be fast, safe, and expressive, making it an excellent choice for developing mobile

17.1 Key Features of Swift

1. Fast and Performant: Swift is designed for performance, offering speed comparable to low-level languages like C. It employs modern techniques like generics, protocol-oriented programming, and value types to optimize code execution.

2. Safe and Secure: Swift emphasizes safety and security. It includes features like strong typing, optional handling, and automatic memory management (ARC) to prevent common programming errors and ensure app stability.

3. Expressive and Concise: Swift provides a clean and expressive syntax that makes code readable and maintainable. It supports modern programming concepts like closures, extensions, and type inference, enabling developers to write more concise and expressive code.

4. Interoperability with Objective-C: Swift is fully interoperable with Objective-C, allowing developers to leverage existing Objective-C libraries and frameworks in their Swift projects. This interoperability enables a smooth transition from Objective-C to Swift and facilitates the integration of legacy code.

5. Strong Ecosystem and Community: Swift benefits from a thriving ecosystem and community. Apple provides comprehensive
documentation, developer tools (Xcode), and resources to support Swift development. The Swift community actively contributes to open-source libraries, frameworks, and tools, expanding the capabilities of the language.

17.2 Getting Started with Swift

1. Installation: To start developing with Swift, you need a Mac running macOS. Install Xcode, Apple's integrated development environment (IDE), from the Mac App Store. Xcode includes the Swift compiler, debugger, and all the necessary tools for app development.

2. Playgrounds: Swift offers a unique feature called Playgrounds, which provides an interactive environment for learning and experimenting with Swift code. Playgrounds allow you to write code and see the results in real-time, making it an excellent tool for beginners to explore Swift concepts.

3. Xcode Projects: To build iOS apps with Swift, you create Xcode projects. Xcode provides a comprehensive set of tools and templates for app development, including interface builders, simulators, and debugging tools.

4. Swift Fundamentals: Before diving into app development, it's essential to learn the fundamentals of Swift. This includes understanding variables, constants, data types, control flow (if-else, loops), functions, classes, and structures.

17.3 Basic Syntax and Concepts

1. Variables and Constants: In Swift, you declare variables using the var keyword and constants using the let keyword. For example:

```
var age = 25
let name = "John"
```

2. Data Types: Swift provides various data types, including integers (Int), floating-point numbers (Double), booleans (Bool), and strings (String). Swift also supports type inference, where the compiler infers the type based on the assigned value.

3. Functions: Functions in Swift are defined using the func keyword, followed by the function name, parameters, and return type. For example:

```
func greet(name: String) -> String {
    return "Hello, \(name)!"
}
```

4. Classes and Structures: Swift supports object-oriented programming through classes and structures. Classes are reference types, while structures are value types. You define classes and structures using the class and struct keywords, respectively.

5. Optionals: Swift uses optionals to handle the absence of a value. An optional represents a variable that can either hold a value or be nil. You declare an optional by appending a question mark (?) to the type. For example:

```
var age: Int? = nil
```

Example: Building a Basic Healthcare App

Let's consider a simple example of building a basic healthcare app in Swift that allows users to track their daily water intake.

```
import SwiftUI
struct WaterIntakeView: View {
    @State private var waterIntake = 0
    var body: some View {
        VStack {
            Text("Daily Water Intake")
                .font(.title)

            Text("\(waterIntake) ml")
                .font(.largeTitle)
```

```swift
                Button(action: {
                  self.waterIntake += 250
                }) {
                  Text("Add 250 ml")
                     .padding()
                     .background(Color.blue)
                     .foregroundColor(.white)
                     .cornerRadius(10)
                }

                Button(action: {
                  self.waterIntake = 0
                }) {
                  Text("Reset")
                     .padding()
                     .background(Color.red)
                     .foregroundColor(.white)
                     .cornerRadius(10)
                }
              }
            }
          }
        }

        struct WaterIntakeView_Previews: PreviewProvider {
          static var previews: some View {
            WaterIntakeView()
          }
        }
```

In this example, we define a WaterIntakeView struct that conforms to the View protocol. The view displays the current water intake and provides buttons to add 250 ml of water and reset the intake.

We use the @State property wrapper to manage the state of the water intake. The body property defines the view's content, which consists of a VStack containing a title, the current water intake, and two buttons.

The "Add 250 ml" button increments the water intake by 250 ml when tapped, while the "Reset" button sets the water intake back to zero.

To preview the view in Xcode, we define a WaterIntakeView_Previews struct that conforms to the PreviewProvider protocol and provides an instance of the

WaterIntakeView.

This example demonstrates the basics of building a user interface and handling user interactions in a Swift app using the SwiftUI framework. SwiftUI provides a declarative way to build user interfaces, making it easier to create responsive and dynamic apps.

Swift's powerful features, combined with its integration with Apple's frameworks like SwiftUI, HealthKit, and Core ML, make it an ideal language for developing mobile healthcare apps. Its focus on safety, performance, and expressiveness enables developers to build robust and efficient apps that can positively impact patient care and engagement

17.4 Developing iOS Apps for Patient Engagement

Patient engagement is a crucial aspect of healthcare, and mobile apps can play a significant role in promoting patient involvement and improving health outcomes. iOS, with its robust ecosystem and user-friendly interface, provides an ideal platform for developing patient engagement apps.

Key Considerations for Patient Engagement Apps:

1. User Experience (UX): Designing an intuitive and user-friendly interface is essential for patient engagement apps. The app should be easy to navigate, visually appealing, and accessible to users with varying technical skills and health literacy levels.

2. Personalization: Incorporating personalization features can enhance patient engagement. This can include customized goals, reminders, and educational content tailored to the patient's specific health condition, preferences, and progress.

3. Gamification: Gamification techniques, such as rewards, badges, and leaderboards, can motivate patients to actively participate in their healthcare. Integrating gamification elements into the app can encourage regular app usage and promote positive health behaviors.

4. Integration with HealthKit: iOS provides a built-in

framework called HealthKit, which allows apps to securely access and share health and fitness data. Integrating with HealthKit enables your app to retrieve relevant health data, such as steps taken, heart rate, and blood glucose levels, to provide personalized insights and recommendations.

5. Data Privacy and Security: Ensuring the privacy and security of patient data is paramount. Implement secure data storage and transmission practices, comply with relevant regulations (e.g., HIPAA), and provide clear privacy policies to build trust with users.

6. Push Notifications: Utilize push notifications to send timely reminders, updates, and encouragement to patients. Notifications can prompt patients to take medications, complete exercises, or attend appointments, helping them stay engaged and adherent to their care plan.

7.Educational Content: Incorporate educational resources, such as articles, videos, and interactive tutorials, to empower patients with knowledge about their health condition, treatment options, and self-management strategies. Providing reliable and accessible information can promote patient engagement and self-care.

8.Communication with Healthcare Providers: Consider integrating features that facilitate communication between patients and their healthcare providers. This can include secure messaging, appointment scheduling, and sharing of health data, enabling patients to actively participate in their care and fostering a strong patient-provider relationship.

Case Study 1: Creating a Medication Adherence App

Medication adherence is a common challenge in healthcare, with many patients struggling to take their medications as prescribed. Let's explore the development of a medication adherence app using Swift and iOS.

Features of the Medication Adherence App:

1. Medication Tracking: Allow users to input and track

their medications, including the name, dosage, frequency, and duration. Provide options to add medication reminders and track adherence over time.

2. Reminders and Notifications: Implement a reminder system that sends push notifications to users at scheduled times, prompting them to take their medications. Include options for customizable reminder settings, such as sound, snooze, and confirmation of medication intake.

3. Adherence Reporting: Generate adherence reports that provide insights into the user's medication-taking behavior. Display visualizations, such as calendars or graphs, to highlight missed doses, adherence patterns, and progress towards goals.

4. Refill Reminders: Incorporate a feature to track medication refills and send reminders when a prescription is running low or approaching its refill date. Integrate with pharmacy APIs, if available, to enable easy refill requests.

5. Educational Content: Provide educational resources related to the user's specific medications, including information about side effects, interactions, and proper administration techniques. Offer tips and strategies for improving medication adherence.

6. Integration with HealthKit: Leverage HealthKit to store and retrieve medication data securely. Integrate with other health data, such as vitals or lab results, to provide a comprehensive view of the user's health status.

7. Caregiver Access: Consider including a feature that allows users to share their medication data with caregivers or family members. This can enable caregivers to monitor adherence, receive alerts, and provide support to the patient.

Implementation Steps:

1. Set up the Xcode project and configure the necessary dependencies and frameworks, such as HealthKit and UserNotifications.

2. Design the user interface using SwiftUI or UIKit, creating intuitive screens for medication input, reminders,

adherence tracking, and educational content.

3. Implement the data models and persistence layer to store medication information securely, utilizing Core Data or a suitable database solution.

4. Integrate with HealthKit to store and retrieve medication data, ensuring proper permissions and data privacy.

5. Implement the reminder system using local notifications or remote push notifications, allowing users to set and customize medication reminders.

6. Develop the adherence tracking and reporting functionality, calculating adherence rates and generating visual representations of medication-taking behavior.

7. Integrate educational content and resources, either by embedding them within the app or by utilizing external APIs or content management systems.

8. Implement caregiver access features, allowing users to securely share their medication data with designated caregivers or family members.

9. Conduct thorough testing and quality assurance to ensure the app's functionality, usability, and performance.

10. Submit the app for App Store review, following Apple's guidelines and requirements for healthcare apps.

One can provide patients with a powerful tool to manage their medications, improve adherence, and engage in their healthcare journey by developing a medication adherence app using Swift and iOS,. The app's features, such as reminders, tracking, and educational content, can empower patients to take control of their medication regimen and promote better health outcomes.

Remember to prioritize data privacy, security, and regulatory compliance throughout the development process. Engage with healthcare professionals, patients, and caregivers to gather feedback and iterate on the app's design and functionality to ensure it meets the needs of its target users.

As you expand the app's capabilities, consider integrating additional features like gamification, social support, and integration with wearable devices to further enhance patient engagement and motivation

Case Study 2: Developing a Symptom Tracking App for Chronic Conditions

Chronic conditions such as diabetes, hypertension, or asthma require regular monitoring and management. A symptom tracking app can help patients keep track of their symptoms, triggers, and health status, enabling better self-management and communication with healthcare providers.

Features of the Symptom Tracking App:

1. Symptom Logging: Allow users to log their symptoms, including the type, severity, and duration. Provide a user-friendly interface for easy and quick symptom entry.

2. Trigger Identification: Enable users to record potential triggers associated with their symptoms, such as diet, exercise, stress levels, or environmental factors. Help users identify patterns and correlations between triggers and symptoms.

3. Health Data Integration: Integrate with HealthKit to access relevant health data, such as blood glucose levels, blood pressure readings, or peak flow measurements, depending on the specific chronic condition.

4. Visualization and Insights: Present symptom and health data in visually appealing charts, graphs, or calendars to help users understand trends and patterns over time. Provide insights and personalized recommendations based on the user's data.

5. Medication Tracking: Incorporate a medication tracking feature that allows users to log their prescribed medications, dosages, and adherence. Provide reminders and alerts for medication intake.

6. Communication with Healthcare Providers: Enable users to share their symptom and health data with their healthcare providers through secure messaging or data export functionality. Facilitate remote monitoring and communication between patients and providers.

7. Educational Resources: Include educational content

specific to the chronic condition, providing users with information about symptom management, lifestyle modifications, and self-care strategies.

Implementation Steps:
1. Set up the Xcode project and configure necessary frameworks like HealthKit and Core Data.
2. Design the user interface for symptom logging, trigger identification, and data visualization screens.
3. Implement data models and persistence for storing symptom, trigger, and medication data securely.
4. Integrate with HealthKit to access and store relevant health data, adhering to privacy and security guidelines.
5. Develop the symptom tracking and visualization functionality, including charts, graphs, and insights generation.
6. Implement medication tracking features, including reminders and adherence tracking.
7. Integrate secure communication channels for sharing data with healthcare providers.
8. Incorporate educational resources and content specific to the chronic condition.
9. Conduct thorough testing and ensure a smooth user experience.
10. Submit the app for App Store review, adhering to healthcare app guidelines.

Case Study 3: Building a Post-Operative Care App for Surgical Patients

Post-operative care is crucial for successful recovery and minimizing complications after surgery. A post-operative care app can provide patients with guidance, reminders, and support during their recovery process.

Features of the Post-Operative Care App:
1. Personalized Recovery Plan: Allow users to input their specific surgery details and generate a personalized recovery plan based on the type of surgery, date, and

healthcare provider's instructions.

2. *Milestone Tracking:* Break down the recovery plan into achievable milestones and allow users to track their progress. Celebrate achievements and provide encouragement along the way.

3. *Wound Care Instructions:* Provide step-by-step instructions and visual aids for proper wound care, including dressing changes, cleaning, and monitoring for signs of infection.

4. *Pain Management:* Include a pain tracking feature where users can log their pain levels, medication usage, and effectiveness. Provide guidance on pain management techniques and when to contact healthcare providers.

5. *Physical Therapy Exercises:* Offer a library of physical therapy exercises tailored to the specific surgery and recovery stage. Provide video demonstrations and instructions for each exercise.

6. *Appointment Reminders:* Integrate with the device's calendar to set reminders for follow-up appointments, physical therapy sessions, and other important post-operative events.

7. *Nutrition and Diet Recommendations:* Provide recommendations for a healthy post-operative diet, including specific guidelines based on the surgery type and any dietary restrictions.

8. *Complication Monitoring:* Educate users about potential post-operative complications and provide a checklist for monitoring signs and symptoms. Include instructions on when to seek medical attention.

Implementation Steps:

1. Set up the Xcode project and configure necessary dependencies.

2. Design the user interface for onboarding, recovery plan creation, milestone tracking, and other key features.

3. Develop data models and persistence for storing personalized recovery plans, progress, and other relevant data.

4. Implement the personalized recovery plan generation based on user input and surgical procedures.

5. Create interactive tracking features for milestones, wound care, pain management, and physical therapy exercises.

6. Integrate with the device's calendar for appointment reminders and notifications.

7. Curate and integrate educational content for nutrition, diet, and complication monitoring.

8. Implement secure data storage and privacy measures
to protect sensitive health information.

9. Conduct thorough testing and ensure the app is user-friendly and accessible.

10. Submit the app for App Store review, following guidelines for healthcare apps.

One can provide patients with a valuable tool to guide them through their recovery process by developing a post-operative care app using Swift and iOS. The app's personalized features, reminders, and educational content can empower patients to actively participate in their own care and improve post-operative outcomes.

Remember to collaborate with healthcare professionals, such as surgeons, nurses, and physical therapists, to ensure the accuracy and relevance of the app's content and features. Continuously gather feedback from users and iterate on the app's design and functionality to meet the evolving needs of post-operative patients.

With a well-designed post-operative care app, you can enhance patient engagement, reduce complications, and support patients in their journey towards successful recovery

18 GO PROGRAMMING FOR SCALABLE HEALTHCARE BACKEND SYSTEMS

Go, also known as Golang, is a modern programming language developed by Google. It is designed to be simple, efficient, and scalable, making it an excellent choice for building backend systems, including those in the healthcare domain. Go combines the simplicity and readability of Python with the performance and concurrency features of low-level languages like C

18.1 Key Features of Go

1. Simplicity and Readability: Go emphasizes simplicity and readability in its syntax and language design. It has a minimal set of keywords and a clean, concise syntax that makes code easy to understand and maintain.

2. *Strong Static Typing:* Go is a statically typed language, which means that variable types are checked at compile-time. This helps catch type-related errors early in the development process and improves code reliability.

3. *Concurrency Support:* Go provides built-in support for concurrency through goroutines and channels. Goroutines are lightweight threads managed by the Go runtime, allowing efficient utilization of system resources. Channels provide a way for goroutines to communicate and synchronize with each other.

4. *Garbage Collection:* Go has an automatic garbage collector that manages memory allocation and deallocation. This relieves developers from the burden of manual memory management and helps prevent common memory-related bugs.

5. *Standard Library and Tooling:* Go comes with a comprehensive standard library that provides a wide range of packages for common tasks, such as networking, file I/O, cryptography, and more. Go also has excellent tooling support, including the go command for building, testing, and managing dependencies.

18.2 Getting Started with Go

1. *Installation:* To start developing with Go, you need to install the Go compiler and tools on your system. Visit the official Go website (https://golang.org) and follow the installation instructions for your operating system.

2. *Go Workspace:* Go uses a specific workspace structure to organize your projects. The workspace typically consists of three directories: src for source code, pkg for compiled package objects, and bin for executable binaries.

3. *Go Modules:* Go uses a dependency management system called Go Modules. It allows you to define and manage dependencies for your projects using the go.mod file. Go Modules ensure reproducible builds and make it easy to share and reuse code.

4. Go Fundamentals: Before diving into backend development, it's essential to learn the fundamentals of Go. This includes understanding variables, data types, control flow (if-else, loops), functions, structs, interfaces, and packages.

18.3 Basic Syntax and Concepts

1. Variables and Constants: In Go, you declare variables using the var keyword, followed by the variable name and type. You can also use the short variable declaration (:=) for inferring the type based on the assigned value. Constants are declared using the const keyword.

```
var age int = 25
name := "John"
const maxValue = 100
```

2. Functions: Functions in Go are defined using the func keyword, followed by the function name, parameters, and return type. Go supports multiple return values.

```
func greet(name string) string {
    return "Hello, " + name + "!"
}
```

3. Structs and Methods: Go uses structs to define custom types that group related data fields. Methods are functions associated with a specific struct type.

```
type Person struct {
    Name string
    Age  int
}

func (p Person) Greet() string {
    return "Hello, my name is " + p.Name
}
```

4. Interfaces: Go interfaces define a set of method signatures. Types that implement all the methods of an interface are said to satisfy that interface. Interfaces provide a way to write flexible and modular code.

```
type Shape interface {
    Area() float64
}
```

```go
type Rectangle struct {
    Width  float64
    Height float64
}

func (r Rectangle) Area() float64 {
    return r.Width * r.Height
}
```

5. *Goroutines and Channels:* Goroutines are lightweight threads that enable concurrent execution. Channels provide a way for goroutines to communicate and synchronize.

```go
func process(ch chan int) {
    // Perform some work
    result := 42
    ch <- result // Send the result to the channel
}
func main() {
    ch := make(chan int)
    go process(ch) // Start a goroutine
    result := <-ch // Receive the result from the channel
    fmt.Println(result)
}
```

18.4 Example: Building a Simple Healthcare API

Let's consider a simple example of building a healthcare API in Go that retrieves patient information.

```go
package main
import (
    "encoding/json"
    "net/http"
)

type Patient struct {
    ID   string `json:"id"`
    Name string `json:"name"`
    Age  int    `json:"age"`
}

var patients = []Patient{
    {ID: "1", Name: "John Doe", Age: 35},
    {ID: "2", Name: "Jane Smith", Age: 28},
}
```

```go
func getPatients(w http.ResponseWriter, r *http.Request) {
    json.NewEncoder(w).Encode(patients)
}

func getPatient(w http.ResponseWriter, r *http.Request) {
    id := r.URL.Query().Get("id")
    for _, patient := range patients {
        if patient.ID == id {
            json.NewEncoder(w).Encode(patient)
            return
        }
    }
    http.NotFound(w, r)
}

func main() {
    http.HandleFunc("/patients", getPatients)
    http.HandleFunc("/patient", getPatient)
    http.ListenAndServe(":8080", nil)
}
```

In this example, we define a Patient struct that represents a patient with an ID, name, and age. We create a slice of Patient instances as sample data.

We define two HTTP handler functions:

getPatients handles the /patients endpoint and returns the list of all patients as a JSON response.

getPatient handles the /patient endpoint and retrieves a specific patient by their ID from the query parameters. If the patient is found, it is returned as a JSON response. Otherwise, a 404 Not Found response is returned.

Finally, in the main function, we register the HTTP handlers using http.HandleFunc and start the server using http.ListenAndServe.

This example demonstrates the basics of building a simple API in Go. In a real-world healthcare backend system, you would typically integrate with databases, handle authentication and authorization, implement more robust error handling, and follow security best practices.

Go's simplicity, performance, and concurrency features make it well-suited for building scalable and efficient healthcare backend systems. Its standard library provides essential packages for web development, database connectivity, and security, making it easier to develop robust and secure healthcare applications.

As you explore Go further, you'll delve into more advanced topics such as concurrency patterns, error handling, testing, and deployment. Go's strong ecosystem and active community provide a wealth of resources, libraries, and frameworks to support your healthcare backend development journey

18.5 Building Microservices and APIs for Healthcare

Microservices architecture has gained significant traction in healthcare software development due to its scalability, flexibility, and modularity. Microservices enable healthcare organizations to develop, maintain, and scale their systems more efficiently by breaking down a monolithic application into smaller, independently deployable services.

18.6 Key Concepts in Microservices Architecture

1. Service Decomposition: Microservices architecture involves decomposing a large application into smaller, loosely coupled services. Each service focuses on a specific business capability or domain, such as patient management, appointment scheduling, or billing.

2. API-Driven Communication: Microservices communicate with each other through well-defined APIs (Application Programming Interfaces). APIs provide a contract for how services interact, enabling loose coupling and independent development of each service.

3. Independent Deployment: Each microservice can be developed, deployed, and scaled independently. This allows for faster development cycles, easier maintenance, and the ability to update or replace individual services without affecting the entire system.

4. Decentralized Data Management: In a microservices architecture, each service typically manages its own data store. This allows services to choose the most suitable database technology for their specific requirements, promoting data autonomy and scalability.

5. *Resilience and Fault Tolerance:* Microservices are designed to handle failures gracefully. Techniques like circuit breakers, retry mechanisms, and load balancing ensure that the system remains resilient and continues to operate even if individual services experience issues.

18.7 Building Microservices in Go

Go is well-suited for building microservices due to its simplicity, performance, and strong support for concurrency. Here are some key considerations when building microservices in Go:

1. *Framework Choice:* Go provides several web frameworks and libraries for building microservices, such as Gin, Echo, and Go kit. Choose a framework that aligns with your requirements and provides the necessary features for building APIs and handling HTTP requests.

2. *API Design:* Design clear and well-documented APIs for your microservices. Use RESTful principles and follow API design best practices, such as using appropriate HTTP methods, status codes, and request/response formats (e.g., JSON).

3. *Service Discovery:* Implement a service discovery mechanism to allow microservices to locate and communicate with each other. Tools like Consul or etcd can be used for service registration and discovery.

4. *Database Integration:* Choose suitable database technologies for each microservice based on its data storage and retrieval requirements. Go provides libraries and drivers for popular databases like PostgreSQL, MySQL, and MongoDB.

5. *Error Handling and Logging:* Implement robust error handling and logging mechanisms in your microservices. Use structured logging libraries like logrus or zap to capture relevant information for debugging and monitoring purposes.

6. *Testing and Continuous Integration:* Write comprehensive

unit tests and integration tests for your microservices. Set up continuous integration and continuous deployment (CI/CD) pipelines to automate the build, test, and deployment processes.

18.8 Case Study 1: Implementing a Distributed Electronic Health Record System

Let's consider a case study of implementing a distributed electronic health record (EHR) system using a microservices architecture in Go.

The EHR system consists of the following microservices:

1. *Patient Service:* Manages patient demographics, medical history, and clinical data.

2. *Appointment Service:* Handles appointment scheduling and management.

3. *Prescription Service:* Manages medication prescriptions and refills.

4. *Billing Service:* Handles billing and insurance-related functionalities.

5. *Reporting Service:* Generates reports and analytics based on patient data.

18.8.1 Implementation Steps:

1. Define the API contracts for each microservice, specifying the endpoints, request/response formats, and any required authentication or authorization mechanisms.

2. Develop each microservice independently using Go and the chosen web framework. Implement the necessary business logic, data storage, and external integrations for each service.

3. Set up a service discovery mechanism, such as Consul, to enable microservices to register themselves and discover other services. This allows services to communicate with each other dynamically.

4. Implement inter-service communication using RESTful APIs or message queues like RabbitMQ or Kafka. Ensure secure communication between services using encryption and authentication protocols.

5. Choose appropriate database technologies for each

microservice based on its data requirements. For example, the Patient Service may use a relational database like PostgreSQL, while the Reporting Service may use a document database like MongoDB for flexible data storage.

6. Implement error handling and logging mechanisms in each microservice. Use structured logging to capture relevant information and centralize logs for easier analysis and debugging.

7. Write comprehensive unit tests and integration tests for each microservice to ensure their correctness and reliability. Use testing frameworks like testing and Ginkgo for writing and running tests.

8. Set up a CI/CD pipeline using tools like Jenkins or GitLab CI/CD to automate the build, test, and deployment processes. Ensure that each microservice is independently deployable and can be scaled based on demand.

9. Deploy the microservices to a container orchestration platform like Kubernetes for efficient management, scaling, and resilience. Use Kubernetes features like deployments, services, and config maps to manage the microservices effectively.

10. Monitor the health and performance of the microservices using monitoring tools like Prometheus and Grafana. Set up alerts and dashboards to proactively identify and resolve any issues.

18.8.2 Benefits of Microservices Architecture in Healthcare

1. Scalability: Microservices allow healthcare systems to scale individual components independently based on demand, ensuring optimal resource utilization and performance.

2. Flexibility: With microservices, healthcare organizations can adapt and evolve their systems more easily. New features or changes can be implemented in specific services without affecting the entire system.

3. Resilience: Microservices are designed to handle failures gracefully. If one service experiences issues, other services can continue to operate, minimizing the impact on the overall system.

4. Technology Diversity: Microservices enable the use of different technologies and frameworks for each service, allowing healthcare organizations to choose the best tools for specific requirements.

5. Faster Development and Deployment: Microservices promote faster development cycles and independent deployments, enabling healthcare organizations to bring new features and improvements to market more quickly.

Implementing a distributed EHR system using a microservices architecture in Go offers several advantages. Go's simplicity, performance, and strong concurrency support make it well-suited for building scalable and efficient microservices.

Healthcare organizations can achieve better scalability, flexibility, and maintainability by decomposing the EHR system into smaller, focused services. Each service can be developed, deployed, and scaled independently, allowing for faster iteration and adaptation to changing requirements.

However, it's important to consider the complexities introduced by microservices, such as distributed data management, inter-service communication, and operational challenges. Proper design, testing, and monitoring are crucial to ensure the reliability and performance of the overall system

18.9 Case Study 2: Building a Real-Time Patient Monitoring System

Real-time patient monitoring systems play a crucial role in healthcare by enabling continuous monitoring of vital signs, alerting healthcare providers to potential issues, and facilitating timely interventions. Let's explore how to build a real-time patient monitoring system using Go and microservices architecture.

The patient monitoring system consists of the following microservices:

1. Device Integration Service: Integrates with various medical devices and sensors to collect real-time patient data, such as heart rate, blood pressure, and oxygen saturation levels.

2. Data Processing Service: Receives the raw data from the Device Integration Service, performs data validation, aggregation, and analysis to derive meaningful insights.

3. Alerting Service: Monitors the processed data from the Data Processing Service and generates alerts based on predefined thresholds or anomaly detection algorithms.

4. Notification Service: Sends notifications and alerts to healthcare providers via various channels, such as mobile push notifications, SMS, or email.

5. Dashboard Service: Provides a real-time dashboard for visualizing patient data, trends, and alerts, enabling healthcare providers to monitor multiple patients simultaneously.

18.9.1 Implementation Steps

1. Design the API contracts for each microservice, specifying the data formats, endpoints, and communication protocols.

2. Develop the Device Integration Service using Go and libraries like gobot or goserial to interface with medical devices and sensors. Implement protocols like HL7 or FHIR for standardized data exchange.

3. Build the Data Processing Service to receive data from the Device Integration Service via messaging queues like Kafka or NATS. Perform data validation, aggregation, and analysis using Go libraries like gonum or gota.

4. Implement the Alerting Service to continuously monitor the

processed data and generate alerts based on predefined rules or machine learning models. Use Go libraries like go-alerts or go-anomaly for alert generation.

5. Develop the Notification Service to send alerts and notifications to healthcare providers. Integrate with services like Twilio for SMS, SendGrid for email, and Firebase Cloud Messaging for mobile push notifications.

6. Create the Dashboard Service using Go web frameworks like Gin or Echo, along with front-end technologies like

React or Vue.js. Visualize real-time patient data using charting libraries like Chart.js or D3.js.

7. Set up a service discovery mechanism like Consul to enable dynamic service registration and discovery. Use gRPC or RESTful APIs for inter-service communication.

8. Implement secure communication between microservices using encryption and authentication mechanisms like SSL/TLS and JSON Web Tokens (JWT).

9. Ensure high availability and fault tolerance by deploying the microservices across multiple nodes and using techniques like load balancing and circuit breakers.

10. Implement comprehensive monitoring and logging using tools like Prometheus and ELK stack to track system health, performance, and troubleshoot issues.

18.9.2 Benefits of Real-Time Patient Monitoring System

1. Early Detection and Intervention: Real-time monitoring enables early detection of potential health issues, allowing for timely interventions and improved patient outcomes.

2. Reduced Manual Monitoring: Automated monitoring reduces the need for manual checks, freeing up healthcare providers' time and minimizing the risk of human error.

3. Centralized Data Access: The dashboard service provides a centralized view of patient data, enabling healthcare providers to monitor multiple patients efficiently.

4. Scalability and Flexibility: Microservices architecture allows for easy scaling of individual components and the ability to add new features or integrate with additional devices seamlessly.

18.10 Case Study 3: Implementing a Telemedicine Platform

Telemedicine platforms have gained significant importance in recent years, enabling remote healthcare consultations and improving access to medical services. Let's explore how to build a telemedicine platform using Go and microservices architecture.

The telemedicine platform consists of the following microservices:

1. *User Management Service:* Handles user registration, authentication, and authorization for patients and healthcare providers.
2. *Appointment Scheduling Service:* Manages appointment scheduling, rescheduling, and cancellations.
3. *Video Consultation Service:* Enables real-time video consultations between patients and healthcare providers using WebRTC technology.
4. *Electronic Health Record (EHR) Service:* Stores and retrieves patient medical records, including consultation notes, prescriptions, and lab results.
5. *Billing and Insurance Service:* Handles billing, invoicing, and insurance claims processing for telemedicine consultations.

Implementation Steps:

1. Design the API contracts for each microservice, specifying the endpoints, request/response formats, and authentication mechanisms.
2. Develop the User Management Service using Go and libraries like jwt-go for authentication and casbin for authorization. Implement secure password hashing and store user information in a database like PostgreSQL.
3. Build the Appointment Scheduling Service to handle appointment creation, rescheduling, and cancellations. Use Go libraries like go-redis for caching and messaging queues like RabbitMQ for event-driven communication.
4. Implement the Video Consultation Service using Go and WebRTC libraries like pion/webrtc. Handle signaling, media streaming, and session management for video consultations.
5. Create the EHR Service to store and retrieve patient medical records. Use a database like MongoDB or CouchDB for flexible and scalable storage. Implement HL7 or FHIR standards for interoperability.
6. Develop the Billing and Insurance Service to generate invoices, process payments, and handle insurance claims. Integrate with payment gateways like Stripe and insurance

APIs for seamless billing and claims processing.

7. Set up a service mesh like Istio or Linkerd to handle service-to-service communication, load balancing, and security. Use gRPC for efficient and type-safe inter-service communication.

8. Implement a API Gateway using Go frameworks like Gin or Echo to provide a single entry point for client applications and handle request routing, authentication, and rate limiting.

9. Ensure data privacy and compliance with regulations like HIPAA by implementing end-to-end encryption, access controls, and audit logging.

10. Implement monitoring and logging using tools like Prometheus, Grafana, and ELK stack to track system performance, identify bottlenecks, and troubleshoot issues.

Benefits of Telemedicine Platform

1. Improved Access to Healthcare: Telemedicine enables patients to access healthcare services remotely, especially in underserved or rural areas.

2. Cost Savings: Telemedicine consultations can be more cost-effective compared to in-person visits, reducing travel and wait times.

3. Convenience and Flexibility: Patients can schedule and attend consultations from the comfort of their homes, saving time and effort.

4. Enhanced Patient Engagement: Telemedicine platforms facilitate better patient engagement through secure messaging, appointment reminders, and access to medical records.

5. Scalability and Extensibility: Microservices architecture allows for easy scaling of individual components and the ability to add new features or integrate with third-party services.

Implementing a telemedicine platform using Go and microservices architecture offers several benefits. Go's simplicity, performance, and concurrency support make it well-suited for building scalable and efficient microservices.

Healthcare organizations can achieve better modularity, scalability, and maintainability by decomposing the telemedicine platform into smaller, focused services. Each service can be developed, deployed, and scaled independently, enabling faster development cycles and easier integration with existing systems.

However, building a telemedicine platform also requires careful consideration of security, privacy, and compliance aspects. Proper encryption, access controls, and audit mechanisms must be implemented to ensure the confidentiality and integrity of patient data.

PART V: EMERGING TRENDS AND FUTURE DIRECTIONS

19 BIG DATA IN HEALTHCARE

The healthcare industry generates a vast amount of data from various sources, including electronic health records (EHRs), medical imaging, genetic sequencing, wearable devices, and social media. This data holds immense potential for improving patient care, optimizing operational efficiency, and driving medical research. However, managing and analyzing such large volumes of complex data poses significant challenges. This is where big data technologies and cloud computing come into play, offering scalable and cost-effective solutions for healthcare data management and analytics

19.1 Big Data in Healthcare

Big data refers to the large, diverse, and complex datasets that are difficult to process and analyze using traditional data processing tools and techniques. In healthcare, big data encompasses structured, semi-structured, and unstructured data from various sources. Some key sources of big data in healthcare include:

1. *Electronic Health Records (EHRs):* EHRs contain patient demographics, medical history, diagnoses, treatments, and medication information. They provide a rich source of structured and unstructured data for analysis.

2. *Medical Imaging:* Medical imaging techniques like X-rays, CT scans, MRIs, and ultrasounds generate large volumes of high-resolution images that require advanced analytics and storage solutions.

3. *Genetic Data:* Advances in genomics and sequencing technologies have led to an explosion of genetic data. Analyzing this data can help in understanding disease risk factors, developing personalized treatments, and identifying drug targets.

4. *Wearable Devices and IoT:* Wearable devices and Internet of Things (IoT) sensors collect real-time data on patient vital signs, activity levels, and environmental factors. This data can be used for remote monitoring, early detection of health issues, and personalized care.

5. *Social Media and Patient-Generated Data:* Social media platforms and online health communities provide valuable insights into patient experiences, sentiments, and behaviors. This data can be used for public health surveillance, patient engagement, and understanding treatment effectiveness.

19.2 Challenges in Healthcare Big Data

While big data offers immense opportunities in healthcare, there are several challenges that need to be addressed:

1. Data Integration and Interoperability: Healthcare data is often siloed across different systems, formats, and standards. Integrating and harmonizing this data is crucial for effective analysis and decision-making.

2. Data Quality and Accuracy: Ensuring the quality and accuracy of healthcare data is essential for reliable insights. Data cleaning, validation, and standardization techniques are required to handle missing, inconsistent, or erroneous data.

3. Data Privacy and Security: Healthcare data contains sensitive personal information that must be protected from unauthorized access and breaches. Compliance with regulations like HIPAA and GDPR is crucial to ensure data privacy and security.

4. Skillset and Expertise: Analyzing healthcare big data requires a combination of domain knowledge, statistical skills, and technical expertise. There is a shortage of professionals with the necessary skillset to leverage big data effectively in healthcare.

5. Computational Resources: Processing and analyzing large volumes of healthcare data requires significant computational resources, including storage, processing power, and bandwidth. Traditional on-premises infrastructure may not be sufficient to handle the scale and complexity of big data.

19.3 Cloud Computing in Healthcare

Cloud computing provides a scalable, flexible, and cost-effective solution for managing and analyzing healthcare big data. Cloud platforms offer on-demand access to computing resources, storage, and analytics tools, enabling healthcare organizations to handle the growing volume and variety of data.

19.3.1 Benefits of Cloud Computing in Healthcare

1. Scalability and Elasticity: Cloud platforms can easily scale up or down based on the data processing and storage requirements. This allows healthcare organizations to handle peak loads and accommodate growing data volumes without significant upfront investments.

2. Cost-Effectiveness: Cloud computing follows a pay-as-you-go model, where organizations only pay for the resources they consume. This eliminates the need for large capital investments in hardware and infrastructure, reducing the total cost of ownership.

3. Data Storage and Accessibility: Cloud platforms provide secure and reliable data storage options, including object storage, data lakes, and data warehouses. Healthcare data can be stored and accessed from anywhere, enabling collaboration and data sharing among healthcare providers, researchers, and patients.

4. Advanced Analytics and Machine Learning: Cloud platforms offer a wide range of analytics tools and machine learning frameworks that can be leveraged for healthcare data analysis. These tools enable predictive modeling, pattern recognition, and data-driven decision-making.

5. Disaster Recovery and Business Continuity: Cloud platforms provide built-in disaster recovery and data backup mechanisms, ensuring the availability and integrity of healthcare data in case of system failures or natural disasters.

19.3.2 Challenges in Healthcare Cloud Adoption

1. Data Security and Privacy: Storing sensitive healthcare data on third-party cloud platforms raises concerns about data security and privacy. Healthcare organizations must ensure that cloud providers adhere to strict security standards and compliance requirements.

2. Regulatory Compliance: Healthcare organizations must comply with various regulations and standards, such as HIPAA, GDPR, and HITECH, when storing and processing data in the cloud. Ensuring compliance requires careful evaluation of cloud provider's security practices and contractual agreements.

3. Data Governance and Control: Moving healthcare data to the cloud may raise concerns about data ownership, control, and governance. Healthcare organizations need to establish clear data governance policies and maintain control over their data assets.

4. Interoperability and Data Integration: Integrating healthcare data from disparate sources and systems in the cloud can be challenging. Standardization efforts and interoperability frameworks are necessary to enable seamless data exchange and integration.

5. Vendor Lock-In: Dependence on a single cloud provider can lead to vendor lock-in, making it difficult to switch providers or migrate data. Healthcare organizations should consider a multi-cloud or hybrid cloud approach to mitigate this risk.

19.3.3 Big Data and Cloud Computing Use Cases in Healthcare

1. Precision Medicine: Analyzing large-scale genomic data, clinical records, and patient-generated data in the cloud enables the development of personalized treatment plans tailored to individual patient characteristics.

2. Population Health Management: Cloud-based big data analytics can help identify high-risk populations, predict disease outbreaks, and optimize resource allocation for improved population health outcomes.

3. Clinical Decision Support: Integrating big data analytics into clinical workflows can provide real-time insights and recommendations to healthcare providers, assisting in diagnosis, treatment selection, and medication management.

4. Remote Patient Monitoring: Cloud-based platforms can collect and analyze real-time data from wearable devices and IoT sensors, enabling remote monitoring of patients, early detection of complications, and timely interventions.

5. Medical Imaging Analytics: Cloud computing provides the computational resources and storage capacity needed to process and analyze large volumes of medical imaging data, enabling advanced image analysis techniques like computer-aided diagnosis and radiomics.

6. Drug Discovery and Development: Cloud-based big data analytics can accelerate drug discovery and development by identifying potential drug candidates, predicting drug efficacy and safety, and optimizing clinical trial design.

Big data and cloud computing are transforming the healthcare industry by providing the tools and infrastructure necessary to manage and analyze vast amounts of complex healthcare data. These technologies offer immense potential for improving patient care, optimizing operational efficiency, and advancing medical research.

However, the adoption of big data and cloud computing in healthcare also poses challenges related to data security, privacy, interoperability, and regulatory compliance. Healthcare organizations must carefully evaluate their data management strategies, choose appropriate cloud platforms, and implement robust security measures to ensure the confidentiality and integrity of patient data.

As the healthcare industry continues to evolve, the integration of big data, cloud computing, and emerging technologies like edge computing, blockchain, and AI will drive further innovation and transformation. Healthcare organizations can unlock the full potential of healthcare data, enabling personalized medicine, improved population health management, and data-driven decision-making by utilizing these technologies.

The future of healthcare lies in the effective utilization of big data and cloud computing to deliver high-quality, patient-centric care while optimizing resource utilization and driving medical research. Healthcare organizations that embrace these technologies and adapt to the changing landscape will be well-positioned to thrive in the era of data-driven healthcare.

20 BLOCKCHAIN APPLICATIONS IN PHARMACY AND MEDICINE

Blockchain technology, originally developed as the underlying infrastructure for cryptocurrencies like Bitcoin, has emerged as a transformative force across various industries, including healthcare. The decentralized, immutable, and transparent nature of blockchain makes it well-suited for addressing several challenges in the pharmaceutical and medical sectors. From drug supply chain management to patient data management and clinical trials, blockchain technology offers a secure and efficient way to streamline processes, improve data integrity, and enhance patient outcomes.

20.1 Understanding Blockchain Technology

Before delving into the specific applications of blockchain in pharmacy and medicine, it is essential to understand the fundamental concepts of this technology.

1. Decentralized Ledger: Blockchain is a decentralized ledger that records transactions across a network of computers. Each participant in the network maintains a copy of the ledger, ensuring transparency and eliminating the need for a central authority.

2. Immutability: Once data is recorded on the blockchain, it cannot be altered or deleted. This immutability ensures the integrity and trustworthiness of the recorded information.

3. Consensus Mechanism: Blockchain networks rely on consensus mechanisms, such as proof-of-work or proof-of-stake, to validate transactions and maintain the integrity of the ledger. These mechanisms ensure that all participants agree on the state of the blockchain.

4. Smart Contracts: Smart contracts are self-executing contracts with the terms of the agreement directly written into code. They automatically enforce the rules and penalties defined in the contract, reducing the need for intermediaries and increasing efficiency.

20.2 Drug Supply Chain Management

One of the most promising applications of blockchain in the pharmaceutical industry is drug supply chain management. The drug supply chain is complex, involving multiple stakeholders, including manufacturers, distributors, wholesalers, and pharmacies. Ensuring the integrity, safety, and authenticity of drugs as they move through the supply chain is a critical challenge.

1. Drug Traceability: Blockchain can enable end-to-end traceability of drugs from the point of manufacture to the point of dispensing. Each transaction in the supply chain can be recorded on the blockchain, creating an immutable and auditable trail. This traceability helps combat counterfeit drugs, prevents diversion, and facilitates recall management.

2. Secure Data Sharing: Blockchain allows secure and controlled sharing of data among supply chain participants. Manufacturers, distributors, and pharmacies can access relevant information, such as product details, batch numbers, and expiration dates, while maintaining data privacy and confidentiality.

3. Regulatory Compliance: Blockchain can help pharmaceutical companies comply with regulatory requirements, such as the Drug Supply Chain Security Act (DSCSA) in the United States. The DSCSA mandates the implementation of an electronic, interoperable system to identify and trace prescription drugs throughout the supply chain.

4. Inventory Management: Blockchain-based solutions can optimize inventory management by providing real-time visibility into drug stocks, reducing the risk of stockouts, and minimizing waste due to expired products.

20.3 Patient Data Management

Managing patient data is another area where blockchain technology can revolutionize healthcare. Electronic Health Records (EHRs) are widely used to store and share patient information, but they often suffer from interoperability issues, data silos, and security vulnerabilities.

1. Decentralized Health Records: Blockchain can enable the creation of decentralized health records, where patients have control over their own data. Patients can grant access to their health information to healthcare providers, researchers, or other authorized parties, ensuring privacy and security.

2. Interoperability: Blockchain-based health records can facilitate interoperability among different healthcare systems and providers. Blockchain can enable seamless data exchange and collaboration, improving care coordination and reducing errors by using standardized data formats and protocols,.

3. Data Security: Blockchain's inherent security features, such as cryptographic hashing and distributed consensus, can enhance the security of patient data. Unauthorized access, tampering, or data breaches can be prevented, protecting sensitive health information.

4. Patient Empowerment: Blockchain-based solutions can empower patients by giving them control over their health data. Patients can track and manage their health records, share data with trusted parties, and participate in research studies, fostering patient-centric care.

20.4 Clinical Trials

Clinical trials are essential for developing new drugs and treatments, but they face challenges related to data integrity, patient recruitment, and confidentiality. Blockchain technology can address these challenges and streamline the clinical trial process.

1. Data Integrity: Blockchain can ensure the integrity and immutability of clinical trial data. All data collected during the trial, including patient information, trial protocols, and results, can be securely recorded on the blockchain, preventing unauthorized modifications or tampering.

2. Patient Recruitment and Consent Management: Blockchain-based platforms can facilitate patient recruitment and consent management for clinical trials. Patients can securely share their health data and provide informed consent through blockchain-based smart contracts, ensuring transparency and accountability.

3. Data Sharing and Collaboration: Blockchain can enable secure data sharing and collaboration among clinical trial stakeholders, such as sponsors, researchers, and regulators. Controlled access to trial data can be granted based on predefined permissions, fostering trust and accelerating the drug development process.

4. Intellectual Property Protection: Blockchain can help protect intellectual property rights associated with clinical trial data and results. Blockchain can prevent unauthorized use or infringement of intellectual property by creating an immutable record of trial data and attributing ownership.

20.5 Prescription Drug Monitoring

Prescription drug abuse and misuse have become significant public health concerns. Blockchain technology can be leveraged to establish a secure and transparent prescription drug monitoring system.

1.*Prescription Tracking:* Blockchain can enable the tracking of prescription drugs from the point of prescribing to the point of dispensing. Each prescription can be recorded on the blockchain, creating an auditable trail and preventing prescription fraud or duplication.

2. *Controlled Substance Monitoring:* Blockchain-based systems can help monitor the distribution and use of controlled substances, such as opioids. Real-time tracking and alerting mechanisms can identify potential abuse patterns and support interventions.

3. *Secure Data Sharing:* Blockchain can facilitate secure data sharing among healthcare providers, pharmacies, and regulatory agencies involved in prescription drug monitoring. Authorized parties can access relevant information while maintaining patient privacy and confidentiality.

4. *Prescription Adherence:* Blockchain-based solutions can help improve prescription adherence by enabling patients to track their medication intake and share data with healthcare providers. Smart contracts can automate refill reminders and adherence incentives, promoting better medication management.

20.6 Challenges and Considerations

While blockchain technology offers numerous benefits in pharmacy and medicine, there are challenges and considerations that need to be addressed for successful implementation.

1. *Scalability:* Blockchain networks need to be scalable to handle the large volumes of data generated in healthcare.

Scalability solutions, such as sharding or off-chain transactions, must be explored to ensure the efficient processing of transactions.

2.Interoperability: Ensuring interoperability among different blockchain platforms and existing healthcare systems is crucial. The development of standards and protocols for data exchange and integration is necessary to realize the full potential of blockchain in healthcare.

3.Regulatory Compliance: The use of blockchain in pharmacy and medicine must comply with existing regulations, such as HIPAA, GDPR, and FDA guidelines. Collaboration between blockchain developers, healthcare organizations, and regulatory bodies is essential to ensure compliance and address legal and ethical considerations.

4. User Adoption: The success of blockchain applications in pharmacy and medicine depends on user adoption. Healthcare providers, patients, and other stakeholders must be educated about the benefits and use cases of blockchain technology. User-friendly interfaces and seamless integration with existing workflows are crucial for widespread adoption.

5. Data Privacy and Security: While blockchain provides inherent security features, additional measures must be implemented to protect sensitive health data. Encryption, access controls, and secure key management are essential to ensure data privacy and prevent unauthorized access.

20.7 Future Outlook

The application of blockchain technology in pharmacy and medicine is still in its early stages, but the potential for transformation is immense. As the technology matures and more use cases are explored, we can expect to see increased adoption and innovation in the healthcare sector.

1. Integration with IoT and Wearables: Blockchain can be integrated with Internet of Things (IoT) devices and wearables to securely collect and store real-time patient data. This integration can enable personalized medicine, remote monitoring, and early detection of health issues.

2. AI and Machine Learning: Combining blockchain with

artificial intelligence (AI) and machine learning can unlock new possibilities in drug discovery, clinical decision support, and predictive analytics. Blockchain can provide secure and auditable data for training AI models, while AI can enhance the efficiency and accuracy of blockchain-based solutions.

3. Personalized Medicine: Blockchain can support the development of personalized medicine by enabling secure and controlled sharing of genomic data, clinical records, and lifestyle information. This data can be used to tailor treatments based on individual patient characteristics, improving treatment outcomes and reducing adverse effects.

4. Global Health Initiatives: Blockchain technology can be leveraged to support global health initiatives, such as disease surveillance, vaccine distribution, and medical supply chain management. Blockchain-based platforms can facilitate secure data sharing and collaboration among international organizations, governments, and healthcare providers, addressing global health challenges.

5. Patient-Centric Ecosystems: Blockchain can enable the creation of patient-centric ecosystems, where patients have control over their health data and can actively participate in their care. Patients can securely share their data with healthcare providers, researchers, and other stakeholders, fostering a more collaborative and personalized approach to healthcare.

The application of blockchain technology in pharmacy and medicine holds immense potential for transforming the healthcare industry. From drug supply chain management to patient data management and clinical trials, blockchain offers a secure, transparent, and efficient way to address longstanding challenges. However, the successful implementation of blockchain in healthcare requires collaboration among stakeholders, addressing scalability and interoperability issues, ensuring regulatory compliance, and promoting user adoption. As the technology evolves and matures, we can expect to see increased innovation and disruption in the pharmaceutical and medical sectors

21 ARTIFICIAL INTELLIGENCE AND DEEP LEARNING IN HEALTHCARE

Artificial Intelligence (AI) and Deep Learning (DL) are transforming various industries, and healthcare is no exception. These technologies have the potential to revolutionize the way we diagnose, treat, and manage diseases, as well as improve patient outcomes and reduce healthcare costs. AI and DL leverage vast amounts of data, advanced algorithms, and computational power to extract insights, make predictions, and assist in decision-making processes. In this chapter, we will explore the applications, challenges, and future prospects of AI and DL in healthcare.

21.1 Fundamentals of AI and Deep Learning

To understand the impact of AI and DL in healthcare, it is essential to grasp the basic concepts behind these technologies.

1. Artificial Intelligence: AI refers to the development of computer systems that can perform tasks that typically require human intelligence, such as visual perception, speech recognition, decision-making, and language translation. AI encompasses various approaches, including machine learning and deep learning.

2. Machine Learning: Machine learning is a subset of AI that focuses on the development of algorithms that can learn from data and improve their performance over time without being explicitly programmed. Machine learning algorithms can be supervised (learning from labeled data) or unsupervised (discovering patterns in unlabeled data).

3. Deep Learning: Deep learning is a subfield of machine learning that uses artificial neural networks with multiple layers to learn hierarchical representations of data. Deep learning models can automatically learn features from raw data, making them particularly suitable for complex tasks such as image recognition and natural language processing.

4. Neural Networks: Neural networks are the building blocks of deep learning. They consist of interconnected nodes (neurons) organized in layers, resembling the structure of the human brain. Each neuron receives inputs, applies a mathematical function, and produces an output that is passed to the next layer. Through training on large datasets, neural networks can learn to make accurate predictions or decisions.

21.2 Applications of AI and Deep Learning in

Healthcare

21.2.1. Medical Imaging and Diagnosis

AI and DL have shown remarkable promise in medical imaging and diagnosis. Deep learning algorithms can analyze medical images, such as X-rays, CT scans, and MRIs, to detect abnormalities, segment anatomical structures, and aid in diagnostic decision-making.

a. Radiology: AI-powered systems can assist radiologists in detecting and classifying various conditions, such as lung nodules, breast lesions, and brain tumors, with high accuracy. These systems can prioritize critical cases, reduce false positives, and improve the efficiency of radiological workflows.

b. Pathology: AI algorithms can analyze digital pathology slides to identify cellular abnormalities, grade tumors, and assist in the diagnosis of diseases like cancer. Deep learning models can learn from large datasets of annotated pathology images, enabling faster and more accurate diagnoses.

c. Ophthalmology: AI-based systems can analyze retinal images to detect signs of diabetic retinopathy, glaucoma, and age-related macular degeneration. These systems can assist in early detection and monitoring of eye diseases, improving patient outcomes and reducing the burden on healthcare providers.

21.2.2. Predictive Analytics and Risk Stratification

AI and DL can analyze large volumes of patient data, including electronic health records (EHRs), genetic information, and lifestyle factors, to predict disease risk, progression, and treatment response.

a. Risk Prediction: AI models can identify patients at high risk of developing certain conditions, such as cardiovascular diseases, diabetes, or sepsis, based on their medical history, vital signs, and other relevant factors. Early identification of at-risk patients allows for proactive interventions and personalized care plans.

b. Readmission Prediction: AI algorithms can predict the

likelihood of patient readmission after hospital discharge by analyzing various factors, such as demographics, comorbidities, and medication history. These predictions can help healthcare providers optimize discharge planning and post-discharge care to reduce readmission rates.

c. Treatment Response Prediction: AI models can analyze patient data to predict the likelihood of treatment response or adverse events. Healthcare providers can make informed decisions and tailor therapies accordingly by identifying patients who are more likely to benefit from a specific treatment or those at higher risk of complications.

21.2.3. Drug Discovery and Development

AI and DL are revolutionizing the drug discovery and development process, accelerating the identification of new drug candidates and improving the efficiency of clinical trials.

a. Virtual Screening: AI algorithms can screen vast libraries of chemical compounds to identify potential drug candidates with desired properties. Deep learning models can learn from molecular structures and predict drug-target interactions, reducing the time and cost associated with traditional drug discovery methods.

b. De Novo Drug Design: AI-powered systems can generate novel drug molecules with specific desired properties, such as efficacy, safety, and bioavailability. These systems can explore the chemical space beyond known compounds, leading to the discovery of innovative drug candidates.

c. Clinical Trial Optimization: AI can analyze historical clinical trial data to identify factors that influence trial success, such as patient selection criteria, dosing strategies, and endpoint definitions. These insights can inform the design of more efficient and targeted clinical trials, reducing costs and accelerating the drug development timeline.

21.2.4. Personalized Medicine

AI and DL enable the development of personalized

treatment approaches tailored to individual patient characteristics, such as genetic profile, medical history, and lifestyle factors.

a. Precision Oncology: AI algorithms can analyze genomic data, imaging features, and clinical information to predict cancer progression, treatment response, and optimal therapy selection. AI can guide personalized cancer treatment strategies by identifying patient-specific tumor characteristics.

b. Pharmacogenomics: AI models can analyze genetic variations to predict drug response and adverse reactions. Healthcare providers can optimize medication selection and dosing, minimizing side effects and improving treatment efficacy by incorporating pharmacogenomic information into treatment decisions.

c. Chronic Disease Management: AI-powered systems can provide personalized recommendations for chronic disease management, such as diabetes, hypertension, and asthma., AI can offer tailored interventions and self-management strategies by analyzing patient data, including self-reported symptoms, sensor readings, and treatment adherence.

21.2.5. Virtual Assistants and Chatbots

AI-powered virtual assistants and chatbots are transforming patient engagement and support in healthcare.

a. Symptom Checkers: AI-based symptom checkers can assist patients in self-assessing their symptoms, providing initial guidance, and recommending appropriate actions, such as seeking medical attention or self-care measures. These tools can help triage patients and reduce unnecessary healthcare visits.

b. Patient Support: AI chatbots can provide personalized patient support, answering common questions, providing educational materials, and assisting with appointment scheduling and medication reminders. These virtual assistants can enhance patient engagement, improve treatment adherence, and reduce the workload on healthcare staff.

c. Mental Health Support: AI-powered conversational agents can offer mental health support, providing empathetic interactions, coping strategies, and resource recommendations. These tools can complement traditional mental healthcare services, increasing access and reducing stigma associated with seeking help.

21.3 Challenges and Considerations

1. Data Quality and Availability: The success of AI and DL in healthcare heavily relies on the availability of high-quality, diverse, and representative datasets. Ensuring data completeness, accuracy, and standardization is crucial for training robust and unbiased models. Addressing data silos, interoperability issues, and privacy concerns is essential for effective AI implementation.

2. Interpretability and Transparency: Many AI and DL models are considered "black boxes," making it difficult to understand how they arrive at specific predictions or decisions. Ensuring interpretability and transparency of AI models is crucial for building trust among healthcare providers and patients. Developing explainable AI techniques and providing clear explanations of model outputs are important considerations.

3. Regulatory and Ethical Considerations: The deployment of AI and DL in healthcare raises regulatory and ethical concerns. Ensuring the safety, efficacy, and fairness of AI-based systems is critical. Regulatory frameworks and guidelines need to be established to govern the development, validation, and deployment of AI in healthcare. Ethical considerations, such as bias mitigation, privacy protection, and informed consent, must be addressed.

4. Integration with Clinical Workflows: Integrating AI and DL solutions into existing clinical workflows can be challenging. Healthcare providers need to be trained on how to use and interpret AI-based tools effectively. Seamless integration with EHR systems, medical devices, and other healthcare technologies is essential for widespread adoption and usability.

5. Liability and Accountability: As AI and DL systems become more involved in healthcare decision-making, questions arise regarding liability and accountability. Clarifying the roles and responsibilities of healthcare providers, AI developers, and other stakeholders is crucial. Establishing legal frameworks and guidelines for AI-related medical errors and adverse events is necessary to ensure patient safety and trust.

21.4 Future Prospects

21.4.1 Continuous Learning and Model Adaptation: AI and DL models have the potential to continuously learn and adapt as new data becomes available. Developing frameworks for real-time model updates and incorporating user feedback can enable AI systems to evolve and improve over time, enhancing their accuracy and relevance in clinical practice.

21.4.2 Federated Learning and Data Privacy: Federated learning is an emerging approach that allows AI models to be trained on decentralized data without the need for data sharing. Federated learning can accelerate AI development in healthcare, particularly in scenarios where data cannot be centralized due to regulatory or confidentiality constraints by enabling collaborative learning while preserving data privacy.

21.4.3 Explainable AI and Interpretability: Research efforts are focused on developing explainable AI techniques that provide clear and understandable explanations of model predictions. Enhancing the interpretability of AI models can increase trust among healthcare providers and patients, facilitating the adoption of AI-based tools in clinical decision-making.

21.4.4 AI-Assisted Robotic Surgery: The integration of AI and robotics in surgical procedures holds immense potential. AI algorithms can analyze surgical videos and provide real-time guidance to surgeons, enhancing precision and minimizing complications. AI-assisted robotic systems can learn from expert surgeons and replicate their techniques, democratizing access to high-quality surgical care.

21.4.5. Wearables and Remote Monitoring: AI and DL can analyze data from wearable devices and remote monitoring systems to provide real-time insights into patient health. AI-powered remote monitoring can improve patient outcomes, reduce hospitalizations, and enable proactive care management by detecting early signs of deterioration, predicting adverse events, and offering personalized interventions.

AI and DL are poised to revolutionize healthcare, offering unprecedented opportunities for improving patient outcomes, optimizing resource utilization, and advancing medical research. From medical imaging and diagnosis to drug discovery and personalized medicine, these technologies have the potential to transform various aspects of healthcare delivery.

However, the successful implementation of AI and DL in healthcare requires addressing challenges related to data quality, interpretability, regulatory compliance, and ethical considerations. Collaboration among healthcare providers, AI researchers, policymakers, and other stakeholders is essential to navigate these challenges and ensure the responsible and beneficial deployment of AI in healthcare.

As AI and DL continue to evolve, we can anticipate further breakthroughs in areas such as continuous learning, federated learning, explainable AI, robotic surgery, and remote monitoring. We can accelerate the transition towards a more personalized, predictive, and proactive healthcare system by harnessing the power of these technologies.

22 QUANTUM COMPUTING AND ITS

POTENTIAL IN HEALTHCARE

Quantum computing, a rapidly evolving field that harnesses the principles of quantum mechanics, is poised to revolutionize various industries, including healthcare. Unlike classical computing, which relies on binary bits (0 or 1), quantum computing utilizes quantum bits (qubits) that can exist in multiple states simultaneously, enabling exponential computational power. This chapter explores the fundamentals of quantum computing and its potential applications in healthcare, discussing the challenges and future prospects of this transformative technology.

22.1 Fundamentals of Quantum Computing

1. Quantum Bits (Qubits): Qubits are the basic unit of quantum information. Unlike classical bits, qubits can exist in a superposition of multiple states (0 and 1) simultaneously. This property allows quantum computers to perform certain computations exponentially faster than classical computers.

2. Quantum Entanglement: Quantum entanglement is a phenomenon where two or more qubits become correlated in such a way that their states are dependent on each other, even when separated by large distances. Entanglement enables quantum computers to perform complex calculations and simulations that are intractable for classical computers.

3. Quantum Algorithms: Quantum algorithms are designed to exploit the unique properties of quantum systems to solve specific problems more efficiently than classical algorithms. Examples include Shor's algorithm for factoring large numbers and Grover's algorithm for searching unstructured databases.

4. Quantum Error Correction: Quantum systems are inherently fragile and prone to errors due to environmental noise and decoherence. Quantum error correction techniques are crucial for maintaining the integrity of quantum computations and enabling reliable quantum computing.

22.2 Potential Applications in Healthcare
22.2.1 Drug Discovery and Development

Quantum computing has the potential to revolutionize drug discovery and development by accelerating the process of identifying novel drug candidates and optimizing their properties.

a. Molecular Simulation: Quantum computers can efficiently simulate complex molecular systems, enabling the accurate prediction of drug-target interactions, binding affinities, and pharmacological properties. This can significantly reduce the time and cost associated with traditional drug discovery methods.

b. Quantum Machine Learning: Quantum machine learning algorithms can analyze vast amounts of molecular data to identify patterns and predict the efficacy and safety of potential drug candidates. Researchers can explore a larger chemical space and identify promising drug leads more efficiently by utilizing the power of quantum computing.

c. Quantum-Assisted Drug Design: Quantum algorithms can aid in the de novo design of drug molecules with desired properties, such as specificity, potency, and bioavailability. Quantum computing can guide the rational design of novel therapeutic agents by exploring the quantum-mechanical properties of molecules.

22.2.2. Personalized Medicine and Genomics

Quantum computing can enable the analysis of massive genomic datasets, facilitating the development of personalized medicine approaches.

a. Quantum Genomic Sequencing: Quantum algorithms can potentially speed up the process of genomic sequencing, enabling the rapid and cost-effective analysis of individual genomes. This can facilitate the identification of genetic variations associated with disease risk, drug response, and treatment outcomes.

b. Quantum-Assisted Precision Medicine: Quantum computing can help integrate and analyze multi-omics data, including genomics, transcriptomics, proteomics, and metabolomics, to generate comprehensive patient profiles. Healthcare providers can tailor personalized treatment plans based on an individual's unique genetic and molecular characteristics by utilizing quantum algorithms.

c. Quantum-Enhanced Genetic Variant Interpretation: Quantum machine learning algorithms can assist in the interpretation of genetic variants, predicting their functional impact and association with disease phenotypes. This can accelerate the identification of clinically relevant variants and guide personalized diagnostic and therapeutic strategies.

22.2.3. Medical Imaging and Diagnostics:

Quantum computing can enhance medical imaging techniques and improve diagnostic accuracy.

a. Quantum Image Processing: Quantum algorithms can efficiently process and analyze medical images, such as MRI, CT, and PET scans. Quantum computers can perform complex image processing tasks, such as segmentation, registration, and feature extraction, with reduced computational time by exploiting quantum parallelism.

b. Quantum-Enhanced Machine Learning for Diagnostics: Quantum machine learning algorithms can be applied to medical imaging data to improve the accuracy of diagnostic models. Researchers can train more sophisticated and efficient machine learning models for disease detection and classification by utilizing the power of quantum computing.

c. Quantum-Assisted Image Reconstruction: Quantum algorithms can aid in the reconstruction of high-quality medical images from incomplete or noisy data. Quantum computing can enable the recovery of missing information and enhance image resolution, leading to improved diagnostic capabilities by exploiting quantum entanglement and superposition.

22.2.4. Quantum Simulation for Disease Modeling

Quantum computing can simulate complex biological systems and disease processes, providing insights into disease mechanisms and potential therapeutic interventions.

a. Quantum Molecular Dynamics: Quantum computers can simulate the dynamic behavior of biomolecules, such as proteins and enzymes, at an atomic level. Researchers can gain a deeper understanding of disease pathways and identify potential drug targets by accurately modeling the interactions and conformational changes of these molecules.

b. Quantum-Assisted Disease Modeling: Quantum algorithms can simulate the progression and spread of infectious diseases, taking into account various factors such as population dynamics, transmission rates, and interventions. These simulations can inform public health strategies and help optimize resource allocation for disease control and prevention.

c. Quantum-Enhanced Systems Biology: Quantum computing can enable the simulation of complex biological networks, such as gene regulatory networks and signaling pathways. Researchers can unravel the underlying mechanisms of diseases and identify potential points of intervention by modeling the intricate interactions and feedback loops within these networks.

22.3 Challenges and Considerations

1. Scalability and Error Correction: Building large-scale, fault-tolerant quantum computers remains a significant challenge. Current quantum devices are limited in the number of qubits and are prone to errors. Overcoming these limitations requires the development of advanced error correction techniques and the scaling up of quantum hardware.

2. Algorithm Development: Designing efficient quantum algorithms that can outperform classical algorithms for specific healthcare applications is a complex task. Researchers need to identify suitable problems that can benefit from quantum speedup and develop tailored quantum algorithms to address these challenges effectively.

3. Data Preparation and Input Encoding: Preparing and encoding classical data into a format suitable for quantum computing is a crucial step. Efficiently mapping healthcare data, such as molecular structures or medical images, onto quantum states requires the development of appropriate encoding schemes and data preprocessing techniques.

4. Integration with Classical Systems: Integrating quantum computing with existing classical healthcare systems and workflows poses challenges. Seamless integration is necessary to leverage the strengths of both quantum and classical computing, enabling a hybrid approach that combines the best of both worlds.

5. Regulatory and Ethical Considerations: The application of quantum computing in healthcare raises regulatory and ethical considerations. Ensuring the safety, privacy, and security of sensitive healthcare data processed by quantum computers is of utmost importance. Establishing guidelines and frameworks for the responsible use of quantum computing in healthcare is crucial.

22.4 Future Prospects

1. Quantum-Assisted Clinical Decision Support: As quantum computing advances, it has the potential to revolutionize clinical decision support systems. Healthcare providers can access real-time, evidence-based recommendations for diagnosis, treatment planning, and patient management by utilizing quantum algorithms and machine learning.

2. Quantum-Enhanced Telemedicine: Quantum computing can enhance telemedicine applications by enabling secure and efficient data transmission, processing, and analysis. Quantum cryptography can ensure the confidentiality and integrity of sensitive medical information exchanged remotely, while quantum algorithms can optimize resource allocation and improve the quality of remote healthcare services.

3. Quantum-Powered Precision Health: The integration of quantum computing with precision health initiatives can accelerate the development of individualized preventive,

diagnostic, and therapeutic strategies. Quantum computers can generate comprehensive health profiles and predict disease risk, enabling proactive and personalized interventions
by analyzing vast amounts of multi-omics data, lifestyle factors, and environmental exposures.

4. Quantum-Assisted Drug Repurposing: Quantum computing can aid in the identification of new therapeutic indications for existing drugs, a process known as drug repurposing. Quantum algorithms can uncover hidden patterns and suggest potential drug candidates for repurposing, accelerating the development of new treatments for unmet medical needs by simulating drug-target interactions and analyzing large-scale biological networks.

5. Quantum-Enhanced Clinical Trials: Quantum computing can optimize the design and execution of clinical trials, improving their efficiency and reducing costs. Quantum algorithms can assist in patient stratification, adaptive trial design, and the prediction of trial outcomes by simulating patient populations. Quantum-assisted clinical trial optimization can accelerate the development and approval of new therapies, bringing innovative treatments to patients faster.

Quantum computing holds immense potential to transform healthcare, offering unprecedented computational capabilities to tackle complex medical challenges. From accelerating drug discovery and personalized medicine to enhancing medical imaging and disease modeling, quantum computing can revolutionize various aspects of healthcare delivery.

However, realizing the full potential of quantum computing in healthcare requires overcoming technical, algorithmic, and integration challenges. Collaboration among quantum computing experts, healthcare professionals, and policymakers is essential to address these challenges and ensure the responsible and effective deployment of quantum computing in healthcare.

240

APPENDICES

A. Useful Libraries and Frameworks for Healthcare Programming

When developing software applications and tools for healthcare, utilizing existing libraries and frameworks can greatly simplify the development process, improve code efficiency, and ensure adherence to industry standards. This appendix provides an overview of some useful libraries and frameworks commonly used in healthcare programming.

1. FHIR (Fast Healthcare Interoperability Resources):
FHIR is a standard for exchanging healthcare information electronically. It defines a set of resources, such as Patient, Observation, and Medication, which can be used to represent and exchange healthcare data.

HAPI FHIR (Java): HAPI FHIR is a Java library that provides a complete implementation of the FHIR specification. It offers tools for parsing, serializing, and validating FHIR resources, as well as a server framework for building FHIR-compliant APIs.

FHIR .NET API (C#): The FHIR .NET API is a .NET library that supports working with FHIR resources in C#. It provides classes for parsing, serializing, and manipulating FHIR resources, as well as a client library for interacting with FHIR servers.

fhir.js (JavaScript): fhir.js is a JavaScript library that enables working with FHIR resources in web applications. It provides utilities for parsing, serializing, and validating FHIR resources, as well as making FHIR API requests from the browser.

2. DICOM (Digital Imaging and Communications in

Medicine)

DICOM is a standard for handling, storing, printing, and transmitting medical imaging information. It defines a file format and network communication protocol for exchanging medical images and related data.

pydicom (Python): pydicom is a Python package for working with DICOM files. It provides tools for reading, writing, and manipulating DICOM data elements, as well as support for DICOM file input/output and dataset handling.

fo-dicom (C#): fo-dicom is a .NET library for working with DICOM files and networks in C#. It offers classes for parsing, creating, and modifying DICOM datasets, as well as support for DICOM network communication and image rendering.

dcmtk (C++): dcmtk is a collection of libraries and applications for reading, writing, and transmitting DICOM files in C++. It provides a comprehensive set of tools for handling DICOM data, including support for DICOM file parsing, network communication, and image conversion.

3. Medical Imaging Libraries

Several libraries are available for processing and analyzing medical images, such as X-rays, CT scans, and MRIs.

SimpleITK (Python, R, Java, C#): SimpleITK is a simplified interface to the Insight Toolkit (ITK), a powerful library for medical image processing. It provides a set of intuitive functions for reading, writing, and manipulating medical images, as well as algorithms for registration, segmentation, and filtering.

NiBabel (Python): NiBabel is a Python package for reading and writing neuroimaging file formats, such as NIfTI, GIFTI, and MINC. It provides a consistent interface for accessing imaging data and metadata, making it easier to work with brain imaging datasets.

MITK (C++): The Medical Imaging Interaction Toolkit (MITK) is a C++ framework for developing interactive medical imaging applications. It offers a wide range of features, including image visualization, segmentation, registration, and tools for building graphical user interfaces.

4. Machine Learning and Deep Learning Frameworks

Machine learning and deep learning techniques have gained significant attention in healthcare for tasks such as disease diagnosis, image analysis, and predictive modeling.

TensorFlow (Python, JavaScript, C++): TensorFlow is an open-source machine learning framework developed by Google. It provides a comprehensive ecosystem for building and deploying machine learning models, including support for deep learning architectures like convolutional neural networks (CNNs) and recurrent neural networks (RNNs).

PyTorch (Python): PyTorch is an open-source machine learning library developed by Facebook. It offers a dynamic computational graph and provides a user-friendly interface for building and training neural networks. PyTorch is known for its flexibility and ease of use, making it popular among researchers and developers.

Keras (Python): Keras is a high-level neural networks API that can run on top of TensorFlow, Microsoft Cognitive Toolkit (CNTK), or Theano. It provides a simple and intuitive interface for building and training deep learning models, abstracting away much of the low-level complexity.

Scikit-learn (Python): Scikit-learn is a popular machine learning library for Python. It provides a wide range of supervised and unsupervised learning algorithms, including support vector machines (SVM), random forests, and k-means clustering. Scikit-learn also offers tools for data preprocessing, model evaluation, and feature selection.

5. Natural Language Processing (NLP) Libraries

NLP techniques are valuable in healthcare for tasks such as clinical text mining, sentiment analysis, and information extraction from unstructured medical records.

NLTK (Python): The Natural Language Toolkit (NLTK) is a popular Python library for NLP tasks. It provides a suite of tools for text preprocessing, tokenization, stemming, part-of-speech tagging, named entity recognition, and more.

NLTK also includes a large collection of corpora and pre-trained
models for various NLP tasks.

spaCy (Python): spaCy is an industrial-strength NLP library for Python. It offers fast and efficient tools for text processing, including tokenization, part-of-speech tagging, dependency parsing, and named entity recognition. spaCy is known for its performance and ease of use, making it suitable for production environments.

Stanford CoreNLP (Java): Stanford CoreNLP is a comprehensive NLP toolkit developed by Stanford University. It provides a set of tools for various NLP tasks, including tokenization, part-of-speech tagging, named entity recognition, coreference resolution, and sentiment analysis. Stanford CoreNLP supports multiple languages and offers a robust set of linguistic annotations.

6. Visualization Libraries

Visualization libraries are essential for presenting healthcare data in a meaningful and interpretable way, enabling researchers and practitioners to gain insights from complex datasets.

Matplotlib (Python): Matplotlib is a fundamental plotting library for Python. It provides a wide range of plotting functionalities, including line plots, scatter plots, bar charts, histograms, and heatmaps. Matplotlib offers fine-grained control over plot customization and is widely used in the scientific community.

Seaborn (Python): Seaborn is a statistical data visualization library built on top of Matplotlib. It provides a high-level interface for creating informative and attractive statistical graphics, such as scatter plots, line plots, bar plots, and violin plots. Seaborn simplifies the process of creating complex visualizations and offers built-in themes for enhancing the aesthetics of the plots.

D3.js (JavaScript): D3.js (Data-Driven Documents) is a powerful JavaScript library for creating interactive and dynamic visualizations in web browsers. It provides a declarative approach to data visualization, allowing developers to bind data to DOM elements and apply data-driven transformations. D3.js offers a wide range of visualization techniques, including charts, graphs, maps, and custom layouts.

7. Bioinformatics Libraries

Bioinformatics libraries are crucial for analyzing and interpreting biological and genomic data in healthcare research.

BioPython (Python): BioPython is a set of freely available tools for biological computation written in Python. It provides modules for handling biological sequences, parsing file formats (e.g., FASTA, GenBank), accessing online databases (e.g., NCBI, ExPASy), and performing common bioinformatics tasks, such as sequence alignment and phylogenetic analysis.

BioPerl (Perl): BioPerl is a collection of Perl modules for bioinformatics. It offers a wide range of functionality, including parsing and manipulating sequence data, accessing databases, performing sequence analysis, and supporting various file formats. BioPerl is widely used in the bioinformatics community and provides a robust framework for developing bioinformatics applications.

Bioconductor (R): Bioconductor is an open-source software project for bioinformatics based on the R programming language. It provides a wide range of tools and libraries for analyzing high-throughput genomic data, including packages for microarray analysis, next-generation sequencing, mass spectrometry, and genomic annotation. Bioconductor is widely used in the bioinformatics research community.

These are just a few examples of the numerous libraries and frameworks available for healthcare programming. The choice of library or framework depends on the specific requirements of the project, the programming language preferences, and the healthcare domain being addressed.

When selecting a library or framework, consider factors such as the level of documentation, community support, licensing, and compatibility with existing systems. It's also important to evaluate the library's performance, scalability, and security features, especially when dealing with sensitive healthcare.

B. Online Resources and Communities for Further Learning

Continuous learning and staying up-to-date with the latest advancements in healthcare programming are essential for professionals in this field. Fortunately, there are numerous online resources and communities available that provide valuable knowledge, practical examples, and opportunities for collaboration. This appendix highlights some of the key online resources and communities that can support further learning and professional growth.

1. Online Courses and Tutorials

Coursera: Coursera offers a wide range of online courses related to healthcare programming, including courses on healthcare data analytics, machine learning for healthcare, and clinical data science. These courses are often taught by industry experts and provide a structured learning experience with video lectures, quizzes, and hands-on projects.

edX: edX is another popular platform for online courses, offering a variety of healthcare-related courses from top universities and institutions worldwide. Courses cover topics such as healthcare informatics, biomedical data science, and health information technology. Many courses are self-paced and offer certificates upon completion.

Udacity: Udacity provides online learning programs, including nanodegree programs focused on healthcare technology. These programs cover topics such as artificial intelligence in healthcare, digital health, and healthcare data analysis. Udacity offers a combination of video lessons, interactive quizzes, and real-world projects to enhance practical skills.

2. Documentation and Tutorials

Official Documentation: The official documentation of libraries, frameworks, and tools used in healthcare programming is an invaluable resource for learning and reference. These documents provide comprehensive guides,

API references, and usage examples. Examples include the FHIR specification documentation, DICOM standard documentation, and documentation for libraries like HAPI FHIR, pydicom, and SimpleITK.

GitHub Repositories: GitHub is a platform where developers share their projects, code snippets, and examples. Many healthcare-related libraries and frameworks have their source code and documentation hosted on GitHub. Exploring these repositories can provide insights into real-world implementations, best practices, and collaborative development.

Blog Posts and Tutorials: Many experienced healthcare programmers and organizations maintain blogs and write tutorials sharing their knowledge and experiences. These resources often provide step-by-step guides, practical examples, and insights into solving specific problems. Examples include the official blogs of healthcare technology companies, as well as personal blogs of industry experts.

3. Online Communities and Forums

Stack Overflow: Stack Overflow is a popular question-and-answer platform for programmers. It has a dedicated healthcare tag where developers can ask questions, seek advice, and share knowledge related to healthcare programming. The community-driven nature of Stack Overflow ensures that answers are peer-reviewed and often provide practical solutions to common problems.

Healthcare-specific Forums: There are several forums and discussion groups specifically focused on healthcare technology and programming. These forums provide a platform for healthcare professionals, developers, and researchers to exchange ideas, seek guidance, and collaborate on projects. Examples include the FHIR community forum, the openEHR forum, and the HL7 discussion groups.

LinkedIn Groups: LinkedIn, a professional networking

platform, hosts various groups related to healthcare technology and programming. Joining these groups allows

professionals to connect with peers, participate in discussions, and stay updated on industry trends and best practices. Examples of relevant groups include "Healthcare Information Technology," "Healthcare Innovation," and "Medical Device Development."

4. Conferences and Webinars

Healthcare Technology Conferences: Attending conferences focused on healthcare technology and programming provides opportunities to learn from industry experts, network with peers, and stay updated on the latest advancements. Some notable conferences include HIMSS (Healthcare Information and Management Systems Society), HL7 FHIR DevDays, and the American Medical Informatics Association (AMIA) Annual Symposium.

Online Conferences and Webinars: With the increasing popularity of virtual events, many conferences and organizations now offer online sessions and webinars. These virtual events allow professionals to attend sessions remotely, access recorded presentations, and engage in live Q&A sessions with speakers. Online conferences and webinars provide a convenient way to learn from experts without the need for travel.

5. Open-source Projects and Collaboration Platforms:

GitHub: GitHub is not only a platform for hosting code repositories but also a hub for open-source projects and collaboration. Many healthcare-related projects, libraries, and frameworks are hosted on GitHub, allowing developers to contribute, report issues, and suggest improvements. Engaging with these projects can provide hands-on experience and opportunities to learn from experienced developers.

GitLab: Similar to GitHub, GitLab is a web-based platform for version control and collaboration. It hosts numerous healthcare-related projects and provides features for issue tracking, continuous integration, and deployment. Participating in GitLab projects can enhance collaboration skills and expose developers to real-world development workflows.

OpenSource EHR and EMR Systems: Several open-source electronic health record (EHR) and electronic medical record (EMR) systems are available, such as OpenEMR and OpenMRS. Contributing to these projects allows developers to gain practical experience in building and maintaining complex healthcare software systems while collaborating with a global community of developers and healthcare professionals.

6. Research Publications and Journals

PubMed: PubMed is a comprehensive database of biomedical literature, including research papers, abstracts, and citations. It covers a wide range of healthcare-related topics, including medical informatics, bioinformatics, and health information technology. Searching PubMed for relevant publications can provide in-depth knowledge and insights into cutting-edge research in healthcare programming.

IEEE Xplore: IEEE Xplore is a digital library that provides access to scholarly articles, conference proceedings, and technical standards published by the Institute of Electrical and Electronics Engineers (IEEE). It includes a significant number of publications related to healthcare technology, biomedical engineering, and health informatics. IEEE Xplore is a valuable resource for staying updated on the latest research and advancements in the field.

Journal of the American Medical Informatics Association (JAMIA): JAMIA is a peer-reviewed journal that focuses on the application of information technology in healthcare. It publishes original research, reviews, and case studies related to various aspects of healthcare informatics, including clinical decision support, electronic health records, and data analytics. JAMIA provides a platform for disseminating high-quality research in healthcare programming and informatics.

7. Social Media and Networking

Twitter: Twitter is a social media platform where healthcare professionals, researchers, and developers share news, insights, and engage in discussions. Following healthcare technology influencers, organizations, and hashtags on Twitter can help professionals stay updated on the latest trends, events, and conversations in the field.

LinkedIn: In addition to joining relevant groups, LinkedIn allows professionals to connect with individuals working in healthcare programming and technology. Building a network of connections can lead to opportunities for collaboration, knowledge sharing, and career advancement.

Slack Communities: Slack is a popular communication platform that hosts various communities and workspaces related to healthcare programming. Joining these communities allows professionals to engage in real-time discussions, seek advice, and collaborate with peers. Examples of healthcare-related Slack communities include "Healthcare.IT" and "HL7 FHIR."

Engaging with these online resources and communities can greatly enhance the learning experience and professional growth of healthcare programmers. It allows individuals to learn from experts, collaborate with peers, and stay updated on the latest advancements and best practices in the field.

However, it's important to exercise caution when participating in online communities and forums. Always verify the credibility of the information shared and be mindful of the potential for misinformation or outdated practices. It's recommended to cross-reference information with official documentation and reputable sources.

C. Real-World Datasets for Practice and Projects

Working with real-world datasets is crucial for healthcare programmers to gain practical experience, develop data analysis skills, and build meaningful projects. This appendix provides an overview of various real-world datasets available for practice and projects in the healthcare domain.

1. MIMIC (Medical Information Mart for Intensive Care)

MIMIC is a widely-used, freely available dataset developed by the MIT Lab for Computational Physiology. It contains de-identified health data associated with over 40,000 patients who stayed in critical care units of the Beth Israel Deaconess Medical Center between 2001 and 2012. The dataset includes demographics, vital signs, laboratory tests, medications, and more. MIMIC is a valuable resource for research in critical care, electronic health records, and clinical decision support systems.

2. UCI Machine Learning Repository - Healthcare Datasets

The UCI Machine Learning Repository hosts a collection of healthcare-related datasets suitable for machine learning and data analysis projects. Some notable datasets include:

Breast Cancer Wisconsin (Diagnostic) Dataset: This dataset contains features computed from digitized images of fine needle aspirates (FNA) of breast mass, aiming to classify tumors as malignant or benign.

Diabetes 130-US Hospitals for Years 1999-2008 Data Set: This dataset represents 10 years of clinical care at 130 US hospitals and integrated delivery networks, focusing on diabetic encounters and patient records.

Parkinson's Disease Classification Data Set: This dataset contains biomedical voice measurements from healthy individuals and those with Parkinson's disease, aiming to classify Parkinson's cases using machine learning techniques.

3. National Health and Nutrition Examination Survey (NHANES)

The National Health and Nutrition Examination Survey (NHANES) is a program of studies designed to assess the health and nutritional status of adults and children in the United States. The dataset includes demographic, socioeconomic, dietary, and health-related information collected through interviews, physical examinations, and laboratory tests. NHANES data is widely used for epidemiological research and public health studies.

4. Medicare Claims Synthetic Public Use Files (SynPUFs)

The Centers for Medicare & Medicaid Services (CMS) provides the Medicare Claims Synthetic Public Use Files (SynPUFs), which contain synthetic beneficiary-level health information. These files are designed to resemble real Medicare data, allowing researchers and programmers to develop and test software applications without compromising the privacy of actual Medicare beneficiaries. SynPUFs include data on beneficiary demographics, inpatient and outpatient claims, prescription drug events, and more.

5. PhysioNet Datasets

PhysioNet is a repository of freely available medical research data, managed by the MIT Laboratory for Computational Physiology. It hosts a wide range of datasets covering various aspects of biomedical signals and clinical data. Some notable datasets include:

MIT-BIH Arrhythmia Database: This dataset contains 48 half-hour excerpts of two-channel ambulatory ECG recordings, annotated with different types of cardiac arrhythmias.

MIMIC Waveform Database: This dataset consists of

thousands of recordings of multiple physiologic signals, including ECG, blood pressure, and respiration, collected from bedside patient monitors in the intensive care unit.

eICU Collaborative Research Database: This dataset contains de-identified health data from over 200,000 admissions to intensive care units across the United States, including vital signs, medications, laboratory measurements, and clinical notes.

6. Kaggle Healthcare Datasets

Kaggle, a popular platform for data science competitions and collaboration, hosts a variety of healthcare datasets contributed by the community. These datasets cover various aspects of healthcare, such as disease prediction, medical imaging, and electronic health records. Some notable datasets include:

COVID-19 Open Research Dataset Challenge (CORD-19): This dataset contains scholarly articles related to COVID-19 and the coronavirus family of viruses, aiming to facilitate research and development of solutions for the pandemic.

RSNA Pneumonia Detection Challenge: This dataset consists of chest X-ray images labeled with the presence or absence of pneumonia, serving as a resource for developing and evaluating pneumonia detection models.

Healthcare Cost and Utilization Project (HCUP) Dataset: This dataset contains inpatient data from multiple states in the United States, including patient demographics, diagnoses, procedures, and cost information.

7. World Health Organization (WHO) Data Repository

The World Health Organization provides a data repository that offers access to various health-related datasets from around the world. These datasets cover topics such as mortality rates, disease incidence, health system indicators, and population health statistics. The WHO data repository is a valuable resource for global health research and comparative analysis.

8. Centers for Disease Control and Prevention (CDC) Data:

The Centers for Disease Control and Prevention (CDC) offers a wide range of health-related datasets and statistics for public use. These datasets cover various aspects of public health, including infectious diseases, chronic conditions, environmental health, and health behaviors. CDC data is commonly used for epidemiological research, public health surveillance, and policy-making.

9. UK Biobank:

UK Biobank is a large-scale biomedical database and research resource containing in-depth genetic and health information from half a million UK participants. The dataset includes extensive phenotypic and genotypic data, such as demographics, lifestyle factors, medical history, imaging scans, and genetic data. UK Biobank is widely used for studying the genetic and environmental determinants of diseases and for advancing personalized medicine research.

10. National Cancer Institute (NCI) Genomic Data Commons:

The National Cancer Institute provides the Genomic Data Commons (GDC), a data sharing platform that contains harmonized cancer datasets from various research programs and projects. The GDC includes data on cancer genomics, clinical information, and biospecimen data. It serves as a valuable resource for cancer research, enabling the development of novel diagnostic and therapeutic approaches.

When working with real-world healthcare datasets, it is crucial to adhere to ethical and legal guidelines for data privacy and security. Many datasets require specific permissions, agreements, or training before access is granted. Researchers and programmers must ensure compliance with relevant regulations, such as HIPAA (Health Insurance Portability and Accountability Act) in the United States or GDPR (General Data Protection Regulation) in the European Union.

It is also important to properly handle missing data, outliers, and data quality issues commonly encountered in real-world datasets. Preprocessing, data cleaning, and appropriate statistical techniques should be applied to ensure the integrity and reliability of the analysis.

Working with real-world datasets provides invaluable experience in dealing with the complexities and challenges inherent in healthcare data. It allows programmers to develop practical skills in data wrangling, feature engineering, and model development. Healthcare programmers can contribute to advancing medical research, improving patient outcomes, and driving innovation in the healthcare industry by utilizing these datasets for practice and projects.

GLOSSARY

This glossary provides definitions for common terms and concepts related to healthcare programming. It serves as a quick reference to help readers understand the terminology used throughout the book.

A

Algorithm: A step-by-step procedure for solving a problem or accomplishing a specific task, often used in the context of computer programming.

API (Application Programming Interface): A set of rules, protocols, and tools that define how software components should interact with each other, enabling communication between different systems or applications.

B

Bioinformatics: An interdisciplinary field that combines biology, computer science, and statistics to analyze and interpret biological data, particularly related to molecular biology and genomics.

Biomedical Data: Data related to health and medical conditions, including patient records, medical images, physiological signals, and genomic information.

C

Clinical Decision Support System (CDSS): A computerized system that assists healthcare professionals in making clinical decisions by providing evidence-based recommendations and alerts based on patient data.

Cloud Computing: The delivery of computing services,

including servers, storage, databases, and software, over the internet (the cloud), enabling scalable and flexible access to resources.

D

Data Analytics: The process of examining and interpreting data to uncover patterns, trends, and insights that can inform decision-making and problem-solving.

Data Interoperability: The ability of different systems and applications to exchange and interpret data seamlessly, ensuring that information can be shared and used effectively across various platforms.

E

Electronic Health Record (EHR): A digital version of a patient's medical history, including demographics, diagnoses, medications, test results, and treatment plans, maintained by healthcare providers.

Encryption: The process of converting sensitive information into a secure, encoded format to protect it from unauthorized access and ensure data confidentiality.

F

Fast Healthcare Interoperability Resources (FHIR): A standard developed by HL7 that defines a set of resources and APIs for exchanging healthcare information electronically, promoting interoperability between different healthcare systems.

G

Genomics: The study of the complete set of genetic information (genome) of an organism, including the structure, function, and evolution of genes.

H

Health Information Exchange (HIE): The secure and electronic sharing of health-related information among healthcare providers, organizations, and patients, enabling better care coordination and informed decision-making.

Health Level 7 (HL7): A set of international standards for the exchange, integration, and retrieval of electronic health information, widely used in healthcare systems to ensure interoperability.

I

Interoperability: The ability of different systems, devices, or applications to connect, communicate, and exchange data seamlessly, without the need for special effort by the user.

J

JSON (JavaScript Object Notation): A lightweight data interchange format that is easy for humans to read and write and easy for machines to parse and generate, commonly used for transmitting data between a server and a web application.

K

Knowledge Base: A centralized repository of information, data, and expertise related to a specific domain or subject area, used to support decision-making, problem-solving, and knowledge sharing.

L

Longitudinal Data: Data collected from the same subjects repeatedly over an extended period, allowing for the analysis of changes and trends over time.

M

Machine Learning: A subset of artificial intelligence that focuses on the development of algorithms and models that enable computers to learn and improve their performance on a specific task without being explicitly programmed.

Medical Imaging: The process of creating visual representations of the interior of the human body for clinical analysis and medical intervention, including techniques such as X-rays, CT scans, MRI, and ultrasound.

N

Natural Language Processing (NLP): A branch of artificial intelligence that deals with the interaction between computers and human language, enabling machines to understand, interpret, and generate human-like text or speech.

O

Ontology: A formal representation of knowledge within a domain, defining concepts, their properties, and the relationships between them, used to facilitate data integration, knowledge sharing, and reasoning.

P

Personalized Medicine: An approach to medical care that tailors treatment and prevention strategies to an individual's unique characteristics, such as their genetic profile, lifestyle, and environment.

Protected Health Information (PHI): Any information about an individual's health status, provision of healthcare, or payment for healthcare that can be linked to a specific person, as defined by HIPAA regulations.

Q

Quality Assurance (QA): The systematic process of checking and verifying that a product or service meets specified requirements and standards, ensuring its reliability, safety, and effectiveness.

R

Real-time Data Processing: The processing of data as it is generated or collected, enabling immediate analysis and actionable insights, often used in monitoring and decision support systems.

S

Semantic Interoperability: The ability of different systems to understand and interpret the meaning of exchanged information in a consistent and unambiguous way, ensuring that data is correctly understood and used across different contexts.

Structured Data: Data that is organized in a predefined format and follows a specific schema, making it easy to search, analyze, and manipulate using computational methods.

T

Telehealth: The delivery of healthcare services and information using telecommunication technologies, such as video conferencing, remote monitoring devices, and mobile applications, enabling remote patient care and consultation.

U

Unstructured Data: Data that does not have a predefined format or organization, often in the form of free text, images, or audio files, requiring specialized processing techniques to extract meaningful information.

Usability: The extent to which a product or system can be used by specified users to achieve specific goals with effectiveness, efficiency, and satisfaction in a given context of use.

V

Validation: The process of ensuring that a system, model, or algorithm performs as intended and meets the specified requirements, often involving testing with known inputs and expected outputs.

Visualization: The representation of data and information in a graphical or pictorial format, enabling users to explore, understand, and communicate complex patterns and relationships more effectively.

W

Wearable Devices: Electronic devices that can be worn on the body, often equipped with sensors and wireless connectivity, used for monitoring health parameters, tracking fitness activities, and providing personalized feedback.

X

XML (eXtensible Markup Language): A markup language that defines a set of rules for encoding documents in a format that is both human-readable and machine-readable, commonly used for data exchange and storage.

Y

YAML (YAML Ain't Markup Language): A human-readable data serialization format that is commonly used for configuration files and data exchange between programming languages.

Z

Zero Trust Security: A security model that assumes no implicit trust and continuously validates every stage of a digital interaction, requiring strict identity verification for every user and device before granting access to resources.

ABOUT THE AUTHORS

Mr. PRAKASH NATHANIEL KUMAR SARELLA

Mr. Prakash Nathaniel Kumar Sarella is an Associate Professor in the Department of Pharmacy at Aditya University, Surampalem, Andhra Pradesh. His research involves innovative drug delivery systems, with a focus on smart packaging systems, oral insulin delivery and cancer therapeutics. He has published over 36 research and review papers in national and international journals

Dr. AVERINENI RAVI KUMAR

Dr. Averineni Ravi Kumar is working as a Professor at Nimra College of Pharmacy in Vijayawada, Andhra Pradesh, India. He has 31 years of experience and has published 106 papers, 15 books, 5 patents and participated in 50 seminars, webinars, and lectures. He is a member of APTI, ABAP, OPF, and IPA.

Ms. GOLLA VENKATA SOWMYASREE

Ms. Golla Venkata Sowmyasree is working as an Assistant Professor in the Department of Pharmaceutics at Annamacharya College of Pharmacy, Rajampet. She completed her PG from Sri Padmavathi Mahila Visvavidyalayam in 2022 and has 1.9 years of teaching experience.

Dr. PAMIDI LAKSHMI PRASANNA

Dr. Pamidi Lakshmi Prasanna is an Assistant Professor of Pharmacy dedicated to teaching and research. Her analytic work utilizes pharmacoinformatics to improve public health outcomes through personalized care and precision medicine. She aims to enhance treatment using real-world data on the safety and effectiveness of drug therapies

Dr. SOUJANYA AKKINENI

Dr. Soujanya Akkineni is an Assistant Professor in the Department of Pharmacy Practice at KVSR Siddhartha College of Pharmaceutical Sciences, Siddhartha Nagar, Vijayawada. She has a total of 5 years work experience including 2 years 4 months of teaching experience and 2 years 6 months experience in Pharma IT sector.

Mrs. CHOLLANGI BHARGAVI

Mrs. Chollangi Bhargavi is an Assistant Professor in the Department of Pharmaceutics at Ranchi College of Pharmacy, Ranchi. She has 3 and a half years of teaching experience and her goal is to equip pharmacy students with necessary skills for a successful career.

Dr. JAYA VASAVI GURRALA

Dr. Jaya Vasavi Gurrala is presently working as an Associate Professor in the Department of Pharmaceutics at SreeBalaji Medical Colleges & Hospitals, Bharath Institute of Higher Education and Research, Chennai, Tamil Nadu. She has published 3 books, 2 book chapters, 5 patents and 13 research & review papers. She has also presented papers and delivered guest lectures at various colleges and forums.

Dr. MEENAKSHI TYAGI

Mrs. Meenakshi Tyagi is an Associate Professor in the Department of Pharmacy at Quantum University, Roorkee. She has 11 years of teaching and research experience and has published 15 research and review papers in various national and international journals.

Dr. V. RAKSHANA

Dr. V. Rakshana is an Assistant Professor in the Faculty of Pharmacy at Bharath Institute of Higher Education and Research. She has hands-on experience in patient care and medication management.

Dr. SYED AFZAL UDDIN BIYABANI

Dr. Syed Afzal Uddin Biyabani is a research scholar at Rajiv Gandhi University of Health Sciences, Bangalore, focusing on newer antidiabetic medications. His research involves comparing the efficacy and safety of SGLT2 and DPP4 inhibitors in patients with type 2 diabetes.

www.ingramcontent.com/pod-product-compliance
Lightning Source LLC
LaVergne TN
LVHW010502200726
843506LV00013B/2494